IMPROVING RESIDENTIAL LIFE FOR DISABLED PEOPLE

IMPROVING RESIDENTIAL LIFE FOR DISABLED PEOPLE

Keith Tully

Brisbane College of Advanced Education
Queensland

Illustrations by John Harrison

Churchill Livingstone

MELBOURNE EDINBURGH LONDON AND NEW YORK 1986

CHURCHILL LIVINGSTONE
Medical Division of Longman Group UK Limited

Distributed in Australia by Longman Cheshire Pty Limited,
Longman House, Kings Gardens, 95 Conventry Street,
South Melbourne 3205, and by associated companies,
branches and representatives throughout the world.

First published 1986
    Reprinted 1989
    Reprinted 1990
    Reprinted 1991

ISBN 0-443-03525-3

British Library Cataloguing in Publication Data
Tully, Keith
    Improving residential life for disabled
    people
    1. Physically handicapped — Institutional
    care
    I. Title
    362.4' 0485   HV3011

Library of Congress Cataloguing in Publication Data
Tully, Keith
    Improving residential life for disabled people.
    Bibliography: p.
    Includes index.
    1. Handicapped — Housing. 2. Housing — Resident
satisfaction. 3. Housing management. I. Title.
[DNLM: 1. Mental Retardation — rehabilitation.
2. Rehabilitation 3. Residential Facilities.
WM 29.1 T923i]
HV1569.T85   1986   362.4' 0485' 068   86-9592

Produced by Longman Singapore Publishers (Pte) Ltd
Printed in Singapore

Preface

Over the past 15 years perceptions of disabled people in most western societies have undergone considerable change. This change has had a significant impact on residential facilities and has led to a critical reappraisal of their relevance for disabled people and their place and function in service provision. As a result, administrators and helpers are today experiencing a great deal of pressure to modify present practices, particularly in relation to definitions of and responses to client need and the quality of residential life.

The major objectives of this book are to summarise what these changes in perceptions mean for residential services and to offer practical ideas for bringing about improvement. The book's content has been oriented to the needs of those physically and intellectually disabled people for whom residential accommodation has, over the past century, been considered the appropriate response. Ideas included have relevance for other forms of residential provision and so may be of value to helpers working with deprived or difficult children, young offenders and frail older people.

It is important that this book is not viewed as a definitive statement on residential provision but as no more than a series of ideas that may be of value when thinking about and attempting to improve present practices. This caution is necessary because there is sometimes a tendency for ideas, once they appear in print, to be viewed as prescriptive. There

will have been considerable bias in the selection of material, despite an attempt to ensure that ideas are consistent with the more progressive approaches to disabled people favoured in many western societies. The need to react critically is implicit in the way the book has been written, and if the manner in which ideas are expressed sometimes suggests to the contrary, that is not intended.

Most helpers employed in residential services are committed to working in ways that benefit disabled people. Present limitations in documented ideas for so doing, however, have resulted in a plea for a kind of recipe book, a document that sets out in clear and concise steps exactly how residential assistance should be provided. While this desire can be understood, there are several reasons why a prescriptive document would be undesirable. First, to be categorical about how disabled people should be assisted is to invest in ideas that, sooner or later, are likely to become out of step with their needs and be a barrier to change. Second, disabled people cannot be viewed and written about as if they were all alike. When perceived as people rather than in terms of their disabilities, they are no more alike than other members of society. Definitions of their needs, and the ways in which they are helped, should be sufficiently flexible to reflect this fact. Third, a basic principle underlying contemporary approaches is that disabled people should be in control of their lives; it follows that any finely detailed and prescriptive statement as to how they should be helped cannot but stand in contradiction to this principle. Fourth, the residences in which disabled people live are immensely varied and at different stages of development. Ideas for the improvement of services should, therefore, be easily adaptable to quite varied situations. Fifth, the process of change in perceptions of and responses to disabled people is not and can never be complete. The way of life of western societies is now based on continuous change, and since attitudes and practices in relation to disabled people are bound up with the values and characteristics of the wider society, responses favoured in the future are unlikely to be the same as those considered appropriate today. For this reason, ideas that purport to suggest better ways of assisting disabled people should not be so definite that they become in themselves a barrier to the development of more enlightened attitudes and approaches.

While the emphasis throughout this book is on the improvement of residential services, there are nevertheless frequent references to traditional ways of perceiving and responding to disabled people. The justification for what may seem a preoccupation with past approaches is that it is difficult to make sense of what is happening today, and constructively plan for tomorrow, without an understanding of the past. More significantly, perhaps, an understanding of the past reveals that many of the attitudes and approaches dominating work with disabled people today are based on quite outdated beliefs and values.

As well as an assumption about the importance of an historical perspective, three other assumptions have influenced selection of material and approach taken. First, an understanding of the way disabled people are perceived and dealt with makes sense only when it is located in an analysis of responses to those groups society defines as deviant. Such an understanding can be attained by use of a sociological perspective, and so sociological concepts feature significantly in the book. Second, conceptions of the needs of disabled people that can best serve their interests should be based on an appreciation of them as members and in the context of the wider society. The conceptual framework for defining need should, therefore, differ from the traditional medical, clinical and casework orientations that have dominated past approaches. Third, the quality of life of disabled people living in residential accommodation is significantly influenced if not determined by organisational factors, particularly the behaviour of those in senior positions. Any suggestions for the improvement of services cannot have much chance of succeeding unless organisational and managerial dimensions are taken into account.

The four parts of this book reflect these assumptions. Part One considers past and present approaches and seeks to provide a framework for the rational and purposeful development of residential services. Part Two looks at ways of identifying and meeting the more important needs of disabled people. Part Three focuses on normalising residential accommodation and Part Four considers a broad range of organisational and management issues. A glossary is included that clarifies terms used in the book, and there is a section containing questions that can be explored when considering the quality of services provided by residential facilities.

K. T.

Contents

ONE

Past and present approaches

Many helpers operate with quite limited understandings of the role and function of residential services. To a great extent this is because the conceptual frameworks they use exclude an analysis of residential care in relation to the wider society, the values from which helpers operate and the nature and distribution of services. As a result, they have little awareness of the influence of social and historical factors on what they do, or of the exaggerated notions of difference on which their conceptions of disabled people are based. Furthermore, the isolated and some-times competitive nature of services suggests there to be little appreciation of the fact that they are provided in a fragmented and irrational way. Finally, since issues relating to intake have warranted little attention, there is scant recognition that many people presently living in the more traditional forms of residential accommodation have no need to be there.

The four chapters that follow seek to redress these conceptual limitations by offering a broad perspective for understanding the nature and function of residential services, and for developing them in ways that are consistent with client need. Chapter 1 looks at the ways disabled people have been perceived and treated until recently, and suggests why it is now necessary to take a quite different approach. Chapter 2 outlines contemporary beliefs about disabled people and the key ideas on which they are based. Chapter 3 explores what is involved in the provision of comprehensive services, and the role of the residential facility, and Chapter 4 looks at issues relating to intake as they apply to residential accommodation.

1

Past approaches to disabled people

This chapter explores responses to disabled people over the past two hundred years and indicates that many of today's services:

- have their origins in the economic and social conditions of early nineteenth century industrialised societies
- reflect definitions of normality and abnormality originating in the nineteenth century
- are built upon negative views of disabled people
- are inconsistent with the nature of late twentieth century society and beliefs about disabled people
- will need to undergo considerable change if better services are to be provided.

RESPONSES IN THE WIDER SOCIAL CONTEXT

There has been a tendency to explain developments in responses to disabled people in somewhat simplistic terms, that is, to view them as a consequence of the efforts of a small number of compassionate and highly motivated individuals. While in some instances this was indeed the case, it is an unsatisfactory explanation of changes over the past two hundred years because it disregards the significance of underlying social factors. Those who influenced approaches to disabled people were responding to problems created and defined by the societies in which they lived. In other words, difficulties that came to be associated with disabled people were a consequence, not of the fact of disability, but of the values and beliefs of mainstream society and the way in which society was organised. This remains no less the case today and any understanding of approaches to disabled people, as well as other minority groups viewed as deviant, should be based on an understanding of the society defining them as, or rendering them, deviant. Specifically, this understanding will be related to the economic and social characteristics upon which the society in question has been structured.

To suggest a relationship between the economic and social characteristics of society and treatment of disabled people may at first seem somewhat surprising. Yet there is a relationship as Figure 1.1 seeks to demonstrate. An analysis such as that conveyed by this chart indicates how:

- different societies define and treat certain groups as deviant
- societies sharing similar social and economic structures define and respond to deviant people in similar ways
- societies with different economic and social structures operate with different conceptions of deviance
- societies experiencing considerable economic and social change will sometimes modify conceptions of what is and what is not deviance, together with ways of responding to deviant people.

ORIGINS OF PRESENT SERVICES

While today's services for disabled people have been influenced by many factors, they are to a considerable extent a consequence of the economic and social conditions prevailing in the nineteenth century. The impact of industrialisation on European and North American countries resulted in major changes in the organisation of social life. As a result, new ways of identifying, defining, and responding to deviant groups came into being.

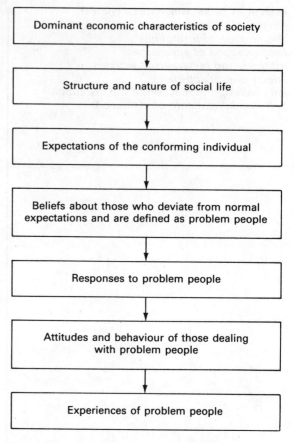

Fig. 1.1 Relationship between the nature of society and responses to problem people.

In exploring approaches over the past two hundred years, this chapter seeks to highlight some of the reasons why disabled people have come to be evaluated and treated in negative ways. Since responses to disabled people have been similar to those of other deviant groups, including the mentally ill, criminals and aged people, much of the discussion is of a generalised nature. The basic argument advanced asserts that because of the characteristics of early industrialised societies and the values on which they were based, those who differed from others in terms of personal attributes or lifestyle could not but be considered as a threat to the well-being of society.

Impact of industrialisation

The radical changes that took place in Europe and North America in the nineteenth century were a consequence of industrialisation. As a result of its impact, society was transformed from a collection of stable, rural communities to large, unstable urban centres. This change in the structure of society destroyed the value system that had bound the small community together and replaced it with new values emphasising quite different notions of social life and of the worth of the individual. As a way of contrasting these changes, Table 1.1 indicates both the characteristics of society prior to and following industrialisation, and the relationship between the nature of a society and its conceptions and treatment of problem people.

Belief systems legitimising industrialisation

These changes were not an inevitable consequence of the invention of machines. In order for mechanised means of production to be adopted to the point of totally restructuring social life, a legitimising social philosophy was essential.

The belief systems that made industrialisation and radical social change possible were the product of liberalism and Protestant theology. Together they propounded the view that individuals were not bound by obligations

Table 1.1 Social change and responses to problem people

	Pre-industrial society	Early industrial society
Dominant economic characteristics of society	Subsistence agriculture and home-based craft industries.	Laissez-faire capitalism; small manufacturing industries; specialised production. Generation of greater production and demand for goods. Wage labour.
Structure and nature of social life	Rigid class system dominated by paternalistic aristocracy and church. Stable rural communities; supportive social networks through parish and extended family.	Authoritarian. Unstable social order as a result of rapid industrialisation and urbanisation. Emphasis on individual effort and competition for survival. Inequality and class system seen as a consequence of personal effort or lack of it. No supportive networks; reliance on nuclear family. Creation of large numbers of paupers.
Expectations of the conforming individual	Should know place and keep to it. Should contribute to community and assist others when capable. Social reciprocity based on Christian teachings that the poor should always be helped.	Responsible for self; should work in order to survive. Should conform to dominant social values. Individual standing in eyes of others assessed in terms of material provision for self and dependents.
Beliefs about those who deviate from normal expectations and are defined as problem people	Origins of much deviance related to external factors. Deviants accepted or tolerated so long as they were not a danger to others. Poor, sick and disabled seen as unfortunates to be assisted by others.	Little differentiation between various groups of deviants; seen as a threat to society; blamed for their condition; had no social usefulness; were a burden on society and so should be excluded.
Responses to problem people	Assisted, to the extent that the community was able, through extended family, parish and Poor Law. Remained psychologically and physically members of society; not judged as inferior.	Punitive approaches aimed at making people more responsible. Those remaining deviant were socially and emotionally isolated, rejected, and, where necessary, removed from society.
Attitudes and behaviour of those dealing with problem people	No special groups of helpers and so no specific set of attitudes and behaviour.	Critical of and hostile to those they dealt with; custodial and controlling role in institutions.
Experiences of problem people	Some ostracism but also much acceptance.	Treated as inferior, in an inhumane way. Tendency to see themselves as others saw them.

to others but were free to act in whatever ways they considered appropriate. It was a short step from such an assertion to the justification of social inequality, competition and exploitation.

Central to such a belief system were new ideas about the value and importance of work both for society and in the life of the individual. In earlier societies work had been accorded little value in itself, it was simply something people did to survive. In contrast, the beliefs supporting industrialisation redefined work and saw it as the most significant dimension of human activity. Being industrious was no longer simply a means to an end but became an end in itself ordained by God. Thus, the greater the efforts of individuals, the greater their spiritual and social fitness and the greater their earthly rewards.

As a consequence of the dominance of this social philosophy, a new set of values regulated social life. Those who worked and provided for themselves and their dependants were viewed as having a right to enjoy the fruits of their labours, whereas those who could not or would not find employment had, at best, a tenuous claim to the means of survival. The minimal help this latter group received was a matter not of entitlement but of charity.

In summary, then, a new set of social values supported rapid industrialisation and urban-isation. In consequence, the social order that had existed for hundreds of years, together with the belief systems on which it had been based, were destroyed. No longer were the notions of social cohesion and reciprocity central to social life. In their place were beliefs emphasising individual action and responsibility. Social fitness became measured by wealth; the unfit were blamed for their condition and expected to suffer the consequences.

Nineteenth century beliefs

The significance placed on individual effort and the value accorded to inequality and competition created hostile and negative attitudes towards those who were unable to work, and those who were at the bottom of the social hierarchy or deviated from it. This negative evaluation was reinforced by other nineteenth century beliefs and concerns such as:

- *fear of over-population* resulting in the view that the lower orders, and particularly problem people, should not be encouraged to propagate
- *the philosophy of utilitarianism* propounding the greatest good for the greatest number, thus implying that, in order for the majority to benefit, there would always be a disadvantaged minority

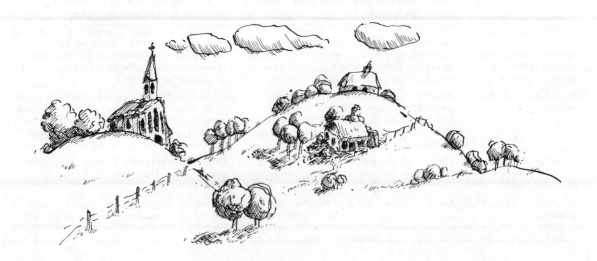

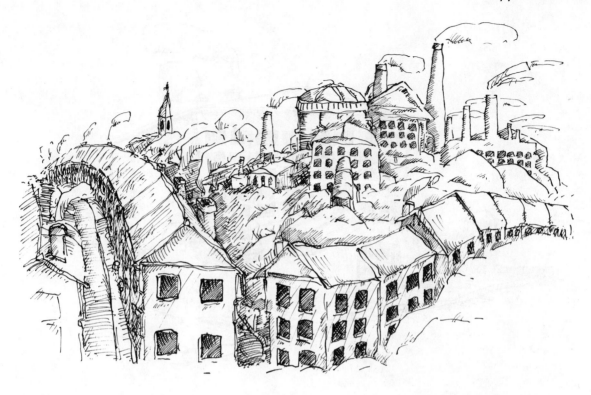

- *the theory of evolution* suggesting it to be natural for only the fittest of a species to survive. It was a simple matter to use such a theory to assert that deviant members of society were unfit and that their survival was against the natural order
- *certain Protestant interpretations of Christianity* arguing that individual well-being or misfortune was explicable only in terms of divine will.

Such a hostile and negative view of social misfits enabled problems and their causes to be projected onto them. Thus they were viewed as:

- having only themselves to blame for their condition
- an insult to the values, beliefs and aspirations of the new social order
- a category of people unwanted by and surplus to the needs of society
- likely to contaminate society by their continued presence
- meriting exclusion from mainstream society.

In the ways in which they were treated, it is evident that most deviant people, regardless of their condition or behaviour, were viewed alike. As has been argued above, disabled people as a category were not differentiated from other social unacceptables and so no special services were developed to care for or assist them.

THE CREATION OF INSTITUTIONS

The destruction of the rural-based social order which had survived for hundreds of years, together with the rapid and chaotic growth in large towns, created chronic instability and a number of threatening social problems. Among such problems were:

- widespread disease as a result of an inadequate supply of fresh water and disposal of sewage and waste matter
- appalling living and working conditions which threatened the continued supply of healthy labour

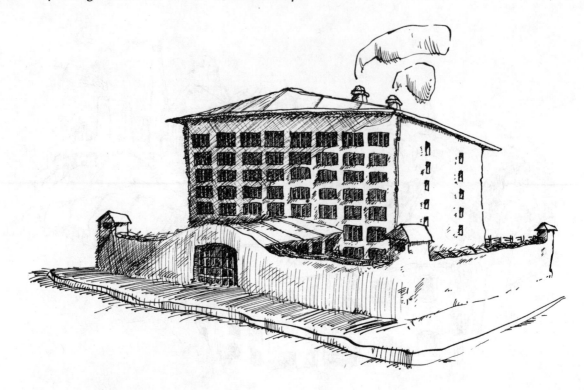

- considerable destitution and poverty as a result of low wages, unemployment, ill-health, disability, infirmity, and the general difficulties of families in caring for their dependent members
- major increase in crime.

Nineteenth century societies set about dealing with such problems in the spirit of cleansing, or sanitising, society by seeking to eliminate all contaminating influences. As far as deviant people were concerned, the favoured solution became the custodial institution. While different solutions could have been developed, the institution was welcomed because it was seen as effectively neutralising those who threatened mainstream society.

The degree of hostility towards those defined as unacceptable can be measured by a willingness to find vast sums of capital for the construction of institutions. From the 1830s many thousands of institutions were planned and built. The first generation of such facilities was in the form of workhouses, initially intended to solve the problems of unemployment and destitution. Later, other facilities were constructed to house specific categories of deviant groups.

By the end of the nineteenth century the construction of institutions throughout the western world resulted in the incarceration and withdrawal from society of hundreds of thousands of children and adults. Into the institution, and often with little discrimination, went destitute children, the incurably sick, the aged, the mentally disturbed and the unemployed and their dependants: all those in fact who could not provide for themselves and had no one else to provide for them.

Influence of the workhouse

The rationale for the construction and mode of operation of workhouses, and particularly British workhouses, was to have considerable influence on the structure and functioning of later institutions, and so it is important to consider why workhouses came into being and what they were meant to achieve.

The British workhouse system was developed as a consequence of the need, identified by the government of the day, to reduce the numbers of unemployed people seeking public assistance. Early nineteenth century society saw itself as incapable of maintaining its unemployed and their dependants and, as a way of denying any responsibility, asserted that unemployment was a voluntary state and self-imposed. Most people, it was argued, could obtain work if they were willing to make sufficient effort. As a way of obliging people to seek work wherever they could and to accept it whatever the rate of pay, the Poor Law Amendment Act of 1834 abolished outdoor relief and made the workhouse the only form of assistance. In order, however, to prevent people remaining in the workhouse and becoming a permanent drain on society, everything about its pattern of life was designed to be so unpleasant that those admitted would strive to leave as soon as they could. In this way the workhouse was meant to act as a strong deterrent to those who might consider seeking public assistance. Furthermore, because of the judgemental attitudes upon which the poor law system was built, it was meant to stigmatise workhouse inmates.

The workhouse system was designed not only to deal with the unemployed but also with other categories of problem people such as orphaned children, the sick and the disabled. While the stated intention was to treat the latter groups in more considerate ways, in practice there was little or no differentiation. All those who through no fault of their own needed help were treated as responsible for their condition.

The workhouse gave way to a later generation of more specialised facilities for the casualities of society in the form of homes, asylums, hospitals and reformatories. In general, despite their various names, most closely resembled the workhouse. In the way these institutions were structured and operated, they were:

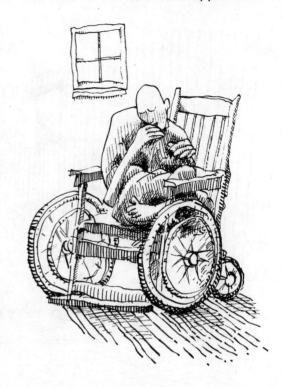

- large, so as to accommodate hundreds and sometimes thousands of inmates on the same site

- assigned a custodial role which was reflected in geographical isolation from community life and in the existence of perimeter walls, fences and other barriers
- given a punitive function which was manifested in dehumanising environments
- seen as self-contained colonies able to meet all basic requirements of inmates, thus eliminating any need for inmates to function in the wider society
- expected to keep the sexes apart
- run as inexpensively as possible resulting in extreme inmate privation and exploitation
- built in a way that necessitated congregate living, with large domitories and day rooms, and communal bathrooms and toilets
- operated in a way that meant the processing of large groups of inmates through every stage of the daily routine
- hostile to any notion of individual need or difference, with inmates simply being viewed as objects to be contained and controlled, given no opportunities for choice or personal decision making, and expected to be compliant, conforming and grateful.

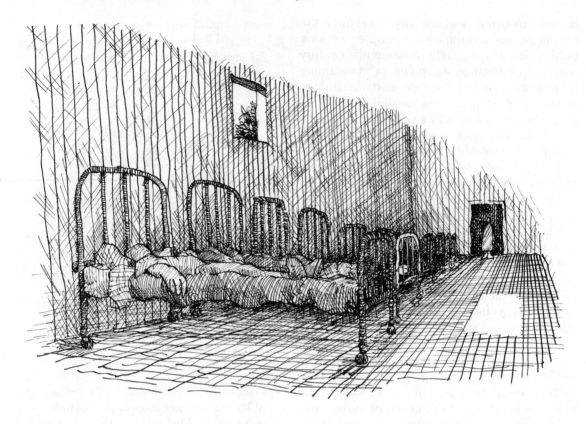

MEDICALISATION OF APPROACHES

The medical and nursing professions were involved in the operation of institutions from the outset, and much of their growth, as well as that of such disciplines as psychology, was a consequence of the growth of institutions.

The use of a medical frame of reference for dealing with deviants was in part a rationalisation for action taken against them. To treat someone who did not conform to accepted social standards as sick was a way of upholding and reinforcing those standards. One of the functions of the institution was to legitimise negative action taken against deviant members of society by acting as bases for the isolation and treatment of those with disabilities and behavioural conditions that were akin to sicknesses.

A major consequence of the medicalisation of responses to deviant people was that many institutions, and particularly those for the disabled, were modelled on the hospital. That meant:

- they were called hospitals

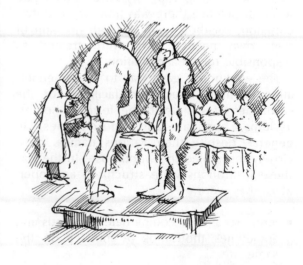

- they were managed and operated by doctors and nurses
- inmates were defined as patients and expected to behave accordingly, that is, to be passive and to co-operate in whatever way was requested of them
- the conforming behaviour demanded of inmates was rationalised in terms of its relevance to a cure and called treatment or therapy
- failure on the part of inmates to conform was seen as a consequence of the pathological nature of their conditions
- living areas were called wards and in design resembled that of the general hospital
- the pattern of life and the daily routine were hospital-like
- the extreme standards of cleanliness and sterile atmosphere associated with the hospital were seen as appropriate for the institution.

Eugenics movement

By the turn of the century most western societies had established extensive systems of institutional care. This was particularly the case in the United States where facilities were viewed as the most progressive in the world. One significant development taken up with considerable enthusiasm in North America, and which served to encourage the growth of the institution and its controlling function for society, was the eugenics movement.

This movement, which was closely allied to medical conceptions of deviant people, was to have consequences for many groups, particularly intellectually and physically disabled people. Its origins can be traced to earlier ideas and beliefs such as the theory of evolution and, to a lesser extent, the concern about too large a population. In relation to the former, it was easy to view disabled people as the unfit members of society who should not survive. It was the eugenics movement that attempted to put such ideas into operation.

At the turn of the century it became popular to believe that most social problems, including ill-health, crime, poverty and intellectual and physical disability, were the direct result of genetic inferiority. In other words, the extent of physical and psychological health and the degree to which individuals could be worthwhile and contributing members of society were related to genetic endowment. Thus, those poorly endowed could not but be a problem to others. Their inferior conditions made them a real threat to social well-being, and because of innate irresponsibility were bound to breed in such profusion as to outnumber and overwhelm the better endowed. The stock of society, therefore, could be maintained only by taking drastic action to eliminate the capacity of the genetically inferior to reproduce.

The ideas of the eugenicists received considerable support in most western societies in the early decades of this century. They were an initial step in a philosophy which culminated in the horrendous actions of fascist Germany in the late 1930s and early '40s. In a less obvious way, and at an earlier point in time, they resulted in the introduction of laws which:

- removed the rights of disabled people as citizens, for example, stripping them of the right to own property
- legalised the collection and retention of many disabled people in custodial institutions
- obliged them to live the whole of their lives with people of their own sex
- defined them as incapables
- prevented them from marrying
- made it possible to sterilise them without their consent.

One by-product of the eugenics movement was the development of concepts and measures of intelligence. The belief that a person's intelligence was fixed at birth and could be measured, provided society with a way of differentiating the fit from the unfit, and this was precisely the use to which intelligence tests at that time were put.

ATTITUDES AND BEHAVIOUR OF WORKERS

The task assigned to the institution was the containment of those people who, for one reason or another, were deemed to merit exclusion from society. As a result, those employed to deal with inmates held negative views of them. The staff role was, in fact, related to the maintenance of good order by demanding inmate compliance to the requirements of the daily routine. This, of course, meant a depersonalising lifestyle for inmates.

In reality, however, those who staffed institutions developed belief systems and rationalisations about their own actions which made what they did appear positive and helpful, and so they sought to deny their custodial role. Nevertheless, most of the practices they developed emphasised and reflected their own needs rather than those of their charges. The needs of staff were, for example, reflected in:

- their hours of work and the way in which duty rosters were structured

- the pattern of daily life that was inflicted on inmates
- forms of control used to deal with those who did not conform
- general limitations imposed upon clients that were contrary to their basic needs
- the superior quality of staff facilities in residences.

EFFECTS OF PAST APPROACHES

From the perspective of disabled people and the reality of life as experienced by them, in addition to having to cope with the personal consequences of disability, they:

- were made to feel guilty for being disabled
- believed themselves to be a burden to society and to their families
- were given a role in society which denied normal interaction with others so that no matter how they behaved or presented themselves, their role reinforced their isolation and difference

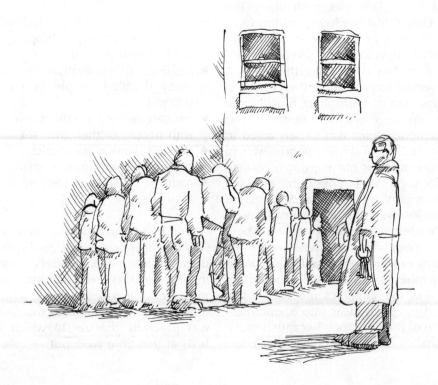

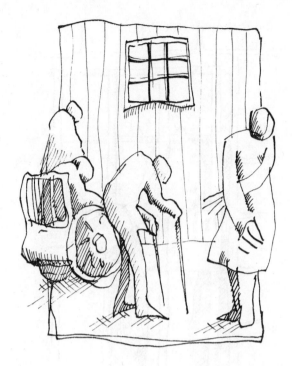

RATIONALISING THE FUNCTION OF THE INSTITUTION

While it is now clear that institutions were constructed to meet society's desire for an effective solution to problems associated with certain categories of deviance, those responsible for establishing and operating such facilities had little awareness of this basic function. They tended to see the institution as having a more positive purpose for society and the deviant individual.

At different times, a number of rationalisations have been favoured for the use of institutions. They have been viewed, for example, as bases for:

- training and rehabilitating those unable to function adequately in society
- providing protection for those incapable of

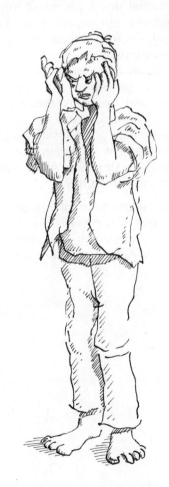

- were punished and stigmatised for being disabled
- were subjected to negligent forms of care which made them abnormal far in excess of any abnormality resulting from disability
- were trapped in a spiral of self-fulfilling prophesy because of conceptions of abnormality held by those closest to them.

Within the institution, this general approach meant:

- experiencing an abnormal and depriving lifestyle
- being forced to share life with others similarly disabled
- being subjected to the dictates of staff
- being denied experiences necessary to build a sense of dignity and worth
- having basic humanness denied by:
  — infantalising lifestyles
  — restricting the development of relationships
  — degrading admission processes designed to shape the person into a typical inmate.

surviving, or likely to be exploited, in a harsh, competitive world, as exemplified in the notion of state as parent and the institution as asylum
- providing effective contexts for meeting the needs of the less fortunate members of society
- treating sick people.

SELF-SUSTAINING NATURE OF INSTITUTIONS

Once institutions had been built they became self-perpetuating because:

- the existence of custodial facilities containing large groups of deviant people served to confirm the need to exclude others like them from society
- the abnormal development of inmates, an unrecognised consequence of inhumane treatment, reinforced their unfitness for life in mainstream society
- the exclusion of so many people resulted in society narrowing its conception of normality and losing its ability to tolerate those who were different
- the attractiveness of the institution prevented the development of alternative forms of help such as those to assist families or based in the community.

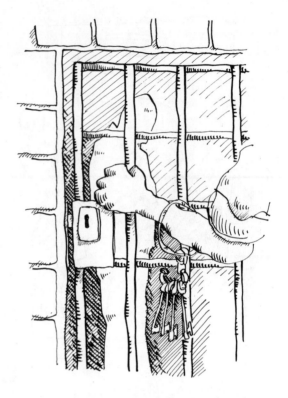

The institutional form of response was so successful that it survived beyond the point where it was consistent with the nature of mainstream society. It was not until the late 1960s that beliefs about problem people, on which the institution has been based, began to be seriously challenged. The outcome of an increasingly critical view of the institution has been an awareness that, as a form of response, it has its origins in and belongs to an earlier society. From the perspective of contemporary society and its beliefs about deviant people, and particularly those who cannot be deemed culpable for their condition, such a response is now seen as punitive and entirely inappropriate.

Contemporary approaches: an overview
Social responses to disability
Contemporary approaches: key ideas

2

Contemporary approaches to disabled people

This chapter explores contemporary approaches to disabled people and the key ideas on which they are based. The approaches discussed, while being quite new, are consistent with the characteristics of present-day society as conveyed by Table 2.1.

In brief, current approaches towards disabled people, in contrast to those which have been dominant until quite recently, advance entirely new ways of:

- perceiving disability and its impact on those who are disabled, their families and the wider society
- conceptualising and responding to need
- providing assistance
- using residential accommodation.

CONTEMPORARY APPROACHES: AN OVERVIEW

Today's approaches are based on the belief that disabled people are qualitatively no different from other members of society. This therefore means that they have an entitlement to a pattern of life and to the rights and freedoms enjoyed by others. Thus there should be an expectation that, unless strong reasons exist to the contrary, they will:

- be nurtured and socialised within the context of the family
- live within mainstream society
- be gainfully occupied on leaving school

15

Table 2.1 Late 20th century society and responses to problem people

Dominant economic characteristics of society	Mixed economy; welfare state. Most employment in large public and industrial organisations
Structure and nature of social life	Democratic and pluralistic. Stable social life. Value placed on quality of life and tolerance of minority groups. Increasing improvements in education, housing, health and welfare
Expectations of the conforming individual	A worthwhile and enjoyable life should be made available to all citizens. Individuals free to live as they see fit, with considerable moral tolerance
Beliefs about those who deviate from normal expectations and are defined as problem people	Judgemental beliefs about those deviating because of their behaviour. Those who deviate through no fault of their own seen as entitled to reasonable assistance
Responses to problem people	Continued negative treatment of offenders. Increasingly positive helping approaches to those who do not conform through no fault of their own; seen as people who should be able to live as others, that is, with independence and in a normal way; basically, the same as everyone else
Attitudes and behaviour of those dealing with problem people	Control the culpable, meet needs of those who cannot be blamed for their condition
Experiences of problem people	Greater tolerance and acceptance. For disabled, increased integration into society

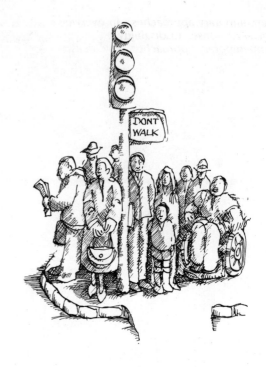

- attain appropriate levels of independence in adulthood
- have opportunities to relate normally to and interact with other members of society.

Possessing a disability can in itself be a barrier to a normal and rewarding life. For most disabled people, development of personal and social competence is dependent upon the provision of adequate services either directly to them or to others involved in their care. In particular, extensive services should be available to families raising disabled children, both in the form of help brought to the home and assistance provided beyond it.

The provision of any service should be seen as an entitlement once a need for it has been identified. From this perspective, help to disabled people is neither a residual welfare function nor dependent upon charitable endeavour. By virtue of their membership of society, disabled people have the right to continuous and effective help in normalised contexts so that the impact and consequences of disability can be minimised. What help they receive should be entirely free from any sense of indebtedness or from stigmatising consequences.

SOCIAL RESPONSES TO DISABILITY

Before exploring some of the more significant ideas on which contemporary approaches are based, it is of value to consider how society responds to the fact of personal impairment. In the past, the existence of a disability was in itself sufficient to warrant an individual's classification in terms of a clearly defined category. While this approach had considerable simplicity, it was unhelpful to disabled people because:

- those identified according to a particular category were perceived uniformly in terms of a stereotype
- the classification systems that existed served to justify segregation from mainstream society
- the significance of mainstream social values in creating negative definitions of disabled people was entirely overlooked
- many disabled individuals capable of normal social functioning were nevertheless perceived in terms of their disability and treated quite differently from other members of society.

The development of new approaches has been accompanied by a search for more helpful ways of identifying those disabled people in need of help. Perhaps one of the most positive attempts, which is reflected in United States' law, stresses that the emphasis should not be on defining people by means of categories and labels, but on recognising the barriers that prevent normal development. From this perspective individuals may be in need of help if they have substantial limitations in one or more of the following areas:

- self care
- receptive and expressive language
- learning
- mobility
- self-direction
- capacity for independent living
- economic sufficiency.

An approach of this kind changes the emphasis from a preoccupation with personal deficits to a focus on individual and environmental factors which inhibit growth and development. One of its consequences is that individuals identified as requiring assistance will not be confined to those in the traditional categories of physical or intellectual disability. Furthermore, those with impairments who are not significantly limited by them should not automatically be defined as in need of specialised assistance.

In summary, then, it makes more sense to recognise the functional consequences of disability than to label a person because of an impairment. With such an approach, disabled people are likely to have their real needs recognised and met and not be perceived and assisted inappropriately.

CONTEMPORARY APPROACHES: KEY IDEAS

Contemporary approaches are expressed in a number of key concepts and ideas. Each serves as a critical comment on past responses as well as being a statement about the orientation and value base for future service provision. The remainder of this chapter considers some of the more significant ideas that have relevance for disabled people and those assisting them. It should be noted that since these ideas have much in common and express the same basic philosophy, there is considerable overlap between them.

In summary, these ideas relate to:

Client rights
Developmental capabilities
Independence and choice
Normalisation and integration
Least restrictive alternative

Client rights

Disabled people have the same basic rights as other members of society as well as the right to services which reduce the impairing effects of their disabilities.

Before exploring what are or should be the rights of disabled people, it is of value to consider why it is necessary to discuss them in the first place. After all, it is not usual to talk in the same way about the rights of those members of society who are not disabled; their rights are so self-evident and are so taken for granted that they only become a point of contention when they are blatantly denied.

The position in regard to disabled people has been somewhat different. As a result of past attitudes and treatment, they have been denied those rights accorded to other

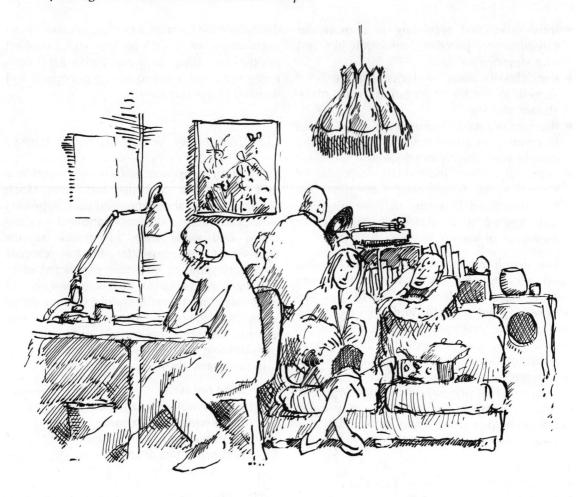

members of society and prevented from asserting them on their own behalf. The fact that the issue of rights is at the centre of contemporary approaches serves to demonstrate past denial of them.

What are rights? There are basically two kinds:

- *legal rights* enacted in and protected by the laws of a society
- *human rights* based upon beliefs about the ways in which human beings should be treated.

Both legal and human rights are founded on four principles:

- all members of society have the same rights. Thus, rights are conferred by citizen-ship, are an entitlement and do not have to be earned
- rights can be limited or denied only as a result of Acts of Parliament or formal decisions by courts of law
- society has an obligation to ensure that the rights of individuals are promoted and protected
- rights impose limitations and responsibilities upon the ways in which members of society behave towards one another.

Today's philosophy asserts that disabled people have the same human value as other members of society and so should not be perceived and treated differently. Their rights, like those of others, are an entitlement, and not something to be given as a reward or denied as a punishment. Thus they cannot be manipulated as if they were a privilege.

The development of approaches towards disabled people is still at the stage where it is necessary to set down some statement about their rights, despite the fact that theirs are no different from others. To suggest what these rights should be will not, of course, guarantee that they will be realised. No list of rights, however comprehensive, is, in itself, more than a statement reflecting the gap between the ideal and the real. It is only when rights are translated into practice and are enforceable that they become a reality in the lives of disabled people.

What are the rights of disabled people? Most statements cover such issues as liberty, growth and maturity, individualisation and independent action. The following list is by no means comprehensive but it does focus upon the more pertinent aspects of the lives of disabled people today. Perhaps it is best viewed as a series of ideas for stimulating discussion of service provision rather than as a static statement of what should be.

Disabled people have the right to:

- *exercise control over their lives*
- *be respected as individuals*
- *liberty*
- *live in the community and, wherever appropriate, with their families*
- *enjoy the moral freedoms of society*
- *grow up and live in environments which, when judged against the standards of society, are normal*
- *be free from personal deprivation and physical harm*
- *freedom of choice, to take risks, and to participate to the fullest extent in all decisions affecting them*
- *assistance which reduces the consequences of disability, which is provided with dignity and humanity, and which recognises them as individuals with unique needs*
- *be assisted by competent and committed staff*
- *have access to all information about themselves.*

Developmental capabilities

Disabled people are capable of growth and development and should experience a pattern of life and receive all necessary assistance that enables them to learn and mature.

The developmental approach is based on the realisation that disabled people have a capacity for growth, development and learning, and for many that capacity is no different from that of other members of society. Helping responses should not, therefore, be built upon beliefs about the dominance and retarding effects of disability but upon identifying the ways in which development can be made possible and enhanced.

Normal growth and development can occur only as a result of:

- positive and intimate relationships with significant others
- normal socialisation experiences
- a pattern of life which includes obligations, incentives and expectations to develop
- fulfilling normal and appropriate roles
- living in normalised settings
- experiencing significant ongoing mainstream social events.

Since a potential for maturation exists in most people, the extent to which it can be realised is not dependent upon personal attributes but upon interactions with others and the context in which those interactions take place. An otherwise normal child, for example, raised in an environment which denies effective socialisation and learning, will become restricted in development.

For those individuals with personal disabilities, the developmental approach suggests that they can develop to the full extent of their capabilities only when their lives are integrated into mainstream society and when all barriers imposed by past practices have been removed. Achieving integration will therefore entail:

- viewing all disabled people as having the potential for growth and development

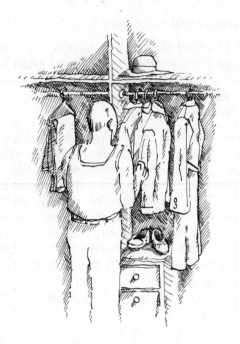

- providing them with experiences to enable development to take place
- encouraging and enabling age-appropriate behaviour.

Approaches based on the developmental model clearly point to the need for effective services and the provision of a normalised lifestyle. Where either is absent, disabled people will be prevented from growing towards maturity.

Any failure to do so cannot be blamed on them but on those who should have provided the appropriate context for development.

Independence and client choice

Disabled people are entitled to exercise control over their lives, to make choices and to become as independent of others as they are able.

The idea of independence in relation to disabled people suggests that they are entitled to control their lives by making their own decisions and choices. While they remain impaired in some way by disability and need help, the assistance they receive should be provided in ways which free them from unreasonable and unnecessary reliance on others.

Independence for disabled people therefore means:

- being able to be responsible for self
- being involved in all decisions affecting self
- being able to acquire and exercise the responsibility that is associated with independent action and choice
- being involved in situations that develop and extend skills for independent action and decision making
- having appropriate freedom of movement
- relating to helpers on the basis of equality and shared responsibility
- being able to express individuality in appearance and other personalised dimensions of life.

To enable disabled people to achieve greater independence helpers in residential accommodation will need to acknowledge that:

- their relationships with clients will differ considerably from those characterising past approaches, particularly in relation to the power they have over clients
- clients have the potential to make their own decisions
- the help they offer should not be so comprehensive that it stifles growth towards maturity and independent behaviour
- their control and support of clients should be reduced if independence is to increase
- independence for the disabled person, like anyone else, is never total; reliance on others in meeting certain basic needs is normal and to be expected
- independent action involves more varied interactions, assertive behaviour and sometimes greater conflict
- difficulties should be resolved, not as a result of arbitrary action on their part, but by processes of negotiation.

Normalisation and integration

The lifestyle of disabled people and the assistance they receive should be consistent with the principle of normalisation.

The principle of normalisation is generally viewed as the most important concept around which to construct appropriate and effective services for disabled people. Whilst it has been the subject of much misunderstanding and misinterpretation, it remains a central idea for identifying present deficiencies in service provision and in shaping new forms of help.

Essentially this concept is a statement about the worth and dignity of those who are disabled. It suggests that disabled people should have available to them the opportunities and conditions for living that are enjoyed by other members of society, so making it possible for them to function as normally as they are able.

Normalisation as an idea represents:

> *A way of life*
> *A basis for the actions of helpers.*

Normalisation as a way of life

Disabled people should be able to:

- follow a normal pattern of development from immaturity to maturity, and not be confined to a child-like and dependent state
- experience a normal yearly cycle, enjoying holidays and seasonal activities as do other people
- experience a normal week, with different arrangements for evenings and weekends when compared with daytime activities from Monday to Friday
- enjoy a normal day, such as being able to get up at a normal hour and attend normal school, work or other daytime activities
- live in as normal a domestic setting as possible
- be able to mix normally in society.

On a practical level normalisation can be pursued and achieved by:

- providing clients with learning experiences that enable them to function more appropriately

- normalising all aspects of the environment in which they live
- ensuring the appearance of clients is not a barrier to integration
- avoiding the use of collective labels
- avoiding services and forms of help which have the consequences of separating clients from others in society, such as special residential, educational, work, leisure and medical arrangements.

It should be noted that normalising the lives of disabled people can never totally remove the impairing effects of many disabilities. A substantial number have disabilities which will restrict them throughout their lives, and this reality should not be denied. There are therefore limits to what can be achieved, but such limits will be identified not as a result of any static and prior assessment, but as an outcome of efforts to increase the developmental potential of clients to enable their lives to be more normal.

In striving to attain normalised lives for disabled people, helpers should realise that:

- the agreement of clients to what happens to them and their participation in decision making processes is, wherever practical, essential

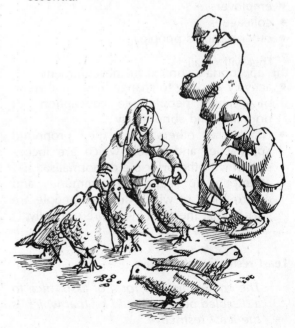

- they should continually be questioning the methods they use in pursuit of the goal of normalisation to satisfy themselves that those methods are ethically acceptable and are not in themselves grossly abnormal
- there are limits to which normalisation for individuals and groups should and can be pursued. Such limits will be determined by the wishes of clients, any inherent limitations imposed by their disabilities or the abnormal nature of a continuous process of trying to bring about change and improvement
- because of the many barriers to be overcome, they may have to make extraordinary efforts to achieve greater normalisation.

Normalisation as a basis for action

Pursuing the goals of normalisation and integration involves helpers not only in providing suitable patterns of life for clients but working for change in the ways disabled people are perceived, defined and treated by:

- the wider society
- the legislature
- government departments
- families
- employers
- colleagues
- other disabled people.

This will entail:

- actively working to change traditional views of disabled people and conceptions of normality and abnormality
- challenging others when they propound approaches and beliefs which are inconsistent with the principle of normalisation
- attempting to shape the community and environment of which disabled people are part so that they can live more normally.

Least restrictive alternative

The context for any form of assistance to a disabled person should be that which is the least restrictive.

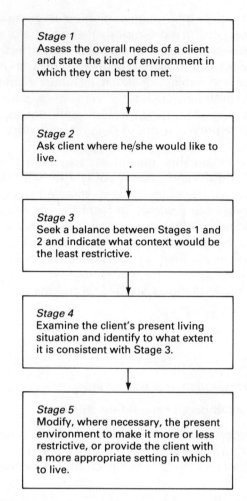

Fig. 2.1 Identifying the least restrictive alternative.

The concept of least restrictive alternative asserts that the context for helping disabled people should be that which is least restrictive in relation to their needs. In other words, an environment or context is the least restrictive when it presents the smallest degree of restraint and disruption to a disabled person's well-being and lifestyle.

The main use of this concept has been related to residential accommodation, suggesting that disabled people should not be removed from their home and community in order to be helped but, wherever possible, services be taken to them at home, made available in their neighbourhood or provided in home-like accommodation in their community. It is, however, an idea that is applicable to other areas of life such as education, health, work and leisure, indicating that these, too, should be pursued in normal social contexts.

The concept of least restrictive alternative, which reflects the high value accorded to human freedom in western societies, began as a legal doctrine in the United States where its prime function was to limit the extent to which government agencies could deprive disabled people of liberty. It is clearly intended as a criticism of custodial forms of care and the unnecessary use of containment and restriction. In operation, it indicates the need to move from services based on large, congregate and restrictive forms of residence to more integrated smaller community based ones.

It is important to be aware that the notion of least restrictive alternative does not assert that all disabled people should live or be assisted in contexts which give them totally unrestricted lives. Because of the nature and extent of some disabilities and certain consequent behavioural difficulties, there will be a small number of disabled people who will require assistance in contexts that impose limitations. The least restrictive alternative for them will not therefore be that which most approximates to the pattern of life enjoyed by mainstream society.

Determining the least restrictive alternative involves achieving a balance between client entitlement on the one hand and their needs and social behaviour on the other. Working through the stages outlined in Figure 2.1 is likely to give a clearer picture of the kind of environment that is appropriate. Any decision about the imposition of restrictions should be taken only where there is compelling evidence that it is necessary for the protection of society or in the interests of a client.

3

Planning services

Existing services for disabled people tend to be unevenly distributed, fragmented and far from comprehensive. As a result, not only is a narrow range of need met, but many clients and their families receive no assistance whatsoever or are obliged to accept forms of help that are inappropriate.

Since contemporary approaches are based on the belief that disabled people are entitled to whatever assistance they need, it is necessary to develop and make available a much broader range of services. Such services are likely to be quite different from those which exist at present because, in being inherited from the past, many of today's services:

- are based on beliefs which are inconsistent with contemporary approaches to disabled people
- bear little relation to identified need
- place a disproportionate emphasis on residential provision
- are generally not particularly helpful to disabled people.

In considering some of the wider issues related to service provision, this chapter:

- suggests the kinds of services which should be made available to disabled people
- argues that specific forms of help may be of little benefit if they are not part of broader rationally-based service plans
- indicates the kind of planning process that may be necessary to achieve comprehensive and co-ordinated services.

It should be recognised that what is described here, were it to be desired, may take many years to attain. In those societies where services for disabled people have developed in a piecemeal fashion as a result of separate initiatives by government, charitable, voluntary and citizen organisations, movement towards planning, rationalisation and development will not be easy. In reality, of course, the provision of comprehensive services is dependent upon certain prior changes, such as:

- greater social, political and profesional awareness of the needs of disabled people
- greater understanding of the factors which disadvantage disabled people
- a willingness on the part of society to allocate an increased proportion of its wealth to meet the needs of its disabled members
- an awareness by organisations at present involved in the delivery of services that change is necessary.

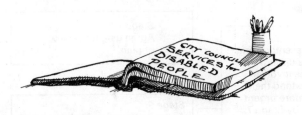

SERVICES: A PLANNING FRAMEWORK

Most services in the past have been provided centrally and this has meant:

- immense variations in access
- geographical mobility of families in search of services for their disabled members, but with the consequent destruction of natural supportive networks
- frequent loss of contact between disabled people and their families where families live some distance from residential facilities
- the virtual impossibility of return to the community for most clients admitted to residential accommodation.

Since the principles underlying contemporary responses suggest a different approach, the planning and delivery of services should be decentralised and regionally organised. In addition to acknowledging the defects associated with centralised services, regionalisation recognises:

- the need for disabled people to be assisted in the context of their families or their natural communities
- that differing regions require planning and service delivery structures reflecting local needs
- that smaller, locally based systems can be more flexible.

The first step in developing comprehensive services will be to create a general awareness that a co-ordinated, rational and overall approach is necessary. Initiatives in this direction can be taken by getting together representatives of service-providing organisations to discuss mutual interests and concerns, and perhaps also to find ways of sharing certain tasks and resources. Considerable time may need to be given to developing the necessary degree of awareness before the next step can be embarked upon.

The second step will be to identify appropriate areas for planning and service delivery. Such areas are likely to be state or county based in the first instance but then, depending upon the population to be served, will be districts of larger cities and regions in less densely populated areas. In whatever way these areas are delineated, they will:

- in cities and towns be sufficiently large in terms of client population to justify a wide range of services, but also small enough to make it possible for clients and their families to travel comfortably to and from home to use community-based forms of help
- in rural communities, be provided by smaller multipurpose organisations offering such services as family counselling and support, and emergency, short-term and longer-term residential care.

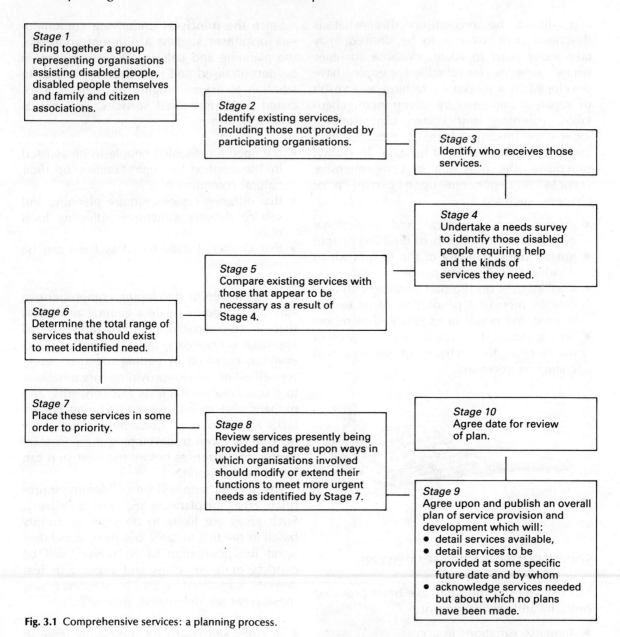

Fig. 3.1 Comprehensive services: a planning process.

The third step will be to embark on a planning process to determine:

- the nature and range of services needed
- how they should be provided
- where they should be based.

The planning process is likely to comprise a series of stages similar to those suggested in Figure 3.1.

Comprehensive service delivery plans, whatever their shape, should be:

- *community based* — within mainstream society
- *decentralised and localised* — as near as possible to the homes of clients
- *comprehensive* — to meet the total range of identified need

- *flexible* — able to be modified when necessary
- *available to all in need* — with no distinction on the basis of race, religion, socio-economic background, ability to pay, etc.
- *rational* — provided only for those whose need has been formally identified
- *continuous* — available for as long as services are needed
- *systematic* — co-ordinated so that there is no unnecessary duplication or gaps in service provision
- *normalised* — consistent with standards implied by the normalisation principle and the notion of least restrictive alternative
- *high quality* — provided by competent helpers
- *dignified* — free from stigma and connotations of charity.

NEEDS ASSESSMENT

The importance of relating service provision to identified need is mentioned frequently throughout this book. Achieving it, however, is far from easy because there is no simple and reliable way of identifying or assessing need.

In the past, the concept of need, if considered relevant at all, tended to be used in a simplistic way. What needs disabled people were seen to have were assessed very narrowly, and generally in relation to the problems they created for others. Thus, quite often, need simply meant need for institutional care. This narrow focus produced groups of professionals with extreme limitations in terms of frames of reference and helping skills. In consequence, professionals assessed the needs of clients in terms of what they could offer and what they considered appropriate. Thus disabled people were identified, for example, as having a need for social work help, for occupational therapy or for psychological testing.

One consequence of the search for new approaches to disabled people has been the extension and development of the concept of need. It is now acknowledged that not only is the process of determining need a complex one but that there are many ways in which need can be assessed, for example:

- clients and their families can be asked to state what they consider their needs to be
- helpers can indicate what they believe the needs of clients to be
- an ideal standard of service provision can be set and need assessed in relation to it
- a minimal standard can be used for need assessment
- need can be assessed in relation to existing service provision or lifestyle, that is, what others, able or disabled, receive or enjoy.

One way of assessing need is not, in itself, better than another. Each approach examines need from a different starting point and so provides different kinds of information. Whenever attempting to assess need it is important to be aware:

- of the conception of need being used and the way it limits and shapes information obtained
- that a comprehensive needs survey will involve a number of approaches including client assessment of need
- that there should not be a great deal of difference between identified needs of clients on the one hand and their acknowledged rights on the other
- that a needs assessment for particular clients and families should be individualised and appropriate to their life situation
- that need is never static but changes over time
- that asking clients and their families to detail their needs, or suggesting that they may have certain needs, raises hopes and expectations about service provision.

SERVICES IN A COMPREHENSIVE PLAN

The total range of services likely to be required by disabled people will be provided by a number of agencies and organisations, including those in the health, education and employment fields. The services detailed below are those which are, for the most part, the responsibility of personal social service organisations. Teams involved in planning services will need to establish links with other bodies so as to achieve some overall integration and consistency in what is offered.

Services directly to parents

- *Counselling*: to help parents understand and cope with the emotional stress and changes in family and social life often associated with having a disabled child
- *information and referral*: including practical guidance relating to the care of disabled children and more general information about the availability of services
- *parent education*: to enable parents to understand, care for and assist their children, and to acquire the ability to act on their own behalf in developing and obtaining services
- *parent support groups*: to act as forums for developing greater understanding and skills, for general sharing of problems, for mutual support, and in establishing pressure groups to seek improvement in services
- *financial and material assistance*: to provide additional resources parents may need to care more effectively for their children.

Services to a family with a disabled relative

Services brought to the home:

- *laundry service*: mainly for those who are incontinent
- *housekeeper/homemaker*: to carry out domestic and other household tasks the carer may not be able to undertake because of time demands in caring for a disabled child or relative
- *personalised help for the disabled individual*: this may involve certain nursing tasks or aspects of personal care such as bathing and exercise

- *a companion service*: to care for disabled people for short periods to enable full-time carers to leave their homes
- *home-based programs*: helpers visit the home to assist in the development of the disabled person's or carer's skills
- *adaptations to the home*: to enable more effective care to take place, for example, installation of a lift or ramp, or provision of a bathroom on the ground floor
- *aids*: a range of aids can be made available, for example, hoists, wheelchairs, toys, special furniture.

Services outside the home:

- *transport*: to enable clients and families to gain access to services, and to make it possible for clients to participate more fully in social life
- *day care*: such as playgroups, nurseries, child minders, adult training centres, day fostering
- *leisure activities*: including individual and group involvement
- *emergency residential care*: in cases of unforseen breakdown in family care
- *overnight care*: on a planned basis to relieve a family
- *short-term relief*: for holiday periods, regular weekday or weekend care
- *longer-term help in residential accommodation*: to achieve certain specified goals detailed in client plans.

Care of children not living with natural parents

- *adoption*: placing a child permanently with others who assume full legal responsibility
- *fostering*: placing a child with others who receive financial payment but who have no legal claims to the child
- *group fostering*: placing a group of children in a fostering setting
- *professional fostering*: paying individuals a direct care worker's salary to care, in their own homes, for severely disabled people, or those whose behaviour is chronically problematic.

Accommodation for disabled adults

- *lodgings*
- *hostels*
- *small community residences*
- *specialised residential facilities*

Services for disabled adults

- *counselling and consultation*
- *laundry service*
- *housekeeper/homemaker*
- *personalised help and personal attendants*
- *home nursing*
- *home-based programs*
- *adaptations to home*

- *aids*
- *financial assistance*
- *transport*
- *employment or other day-time occupation*
- *day care*
- *rehabilitation services*
- *emergency residential care*
- *leisure activities*

SERVICE PROVISION: ROLE OF RESIDENTIAL ACCOMMODATION

The range of services likely to be included in a comprehensive service plan suggests a need for a variety of residential facilities whose

Table 3.1 Range of residential accommodation

Reasons for provision of residential assistance	Timescale	Kinds of assistance needed	Type of facility
Provision of home	Short or longer term or permanent	Normalised daily life; needs met according to individual plan	Appropriate to client's needs
Family support: • illness • emergency • ongoing regular relief	Short term, governed by clear contract	High quality nurturing; normal pattern of daily life; home-like environment; close contact with family, with necessary specialist support	Small locally-based resource
Holiday	Short term, governed by clear contract	Stimulating, different: opportunities for doing new things	Resource in attractive coastal or inland location
Relief of deteriorating situations	Short, longer term or permanent	Normalised daily life; needs met according to individual plan. Close contact with family or caring situation	Appropriate to client's needs
Removal fron unsatisfactory situation	Short or longer term; subject to assessment of client's needs, home situation and alternative forms of care	Normalised daily life; assessment; individual planning to identify needs and decide best course of action. Close contact with family or caring situation	Locally-based facility with necessary resources and staff
Assessment and investigation	Short term, governed by clear contract	Normalised daily life; assessment and evaluation of client's needs leading to formal conference to determine how these needs should be met	Facility with appropriate resources and staff capable of undertaking necessary assessment
Development of client skills, e.g. self-care community survival and integration	Short term, governed by clear contract	Normalised daily life; individual planning and effective programming	Locally-based facility with necessary resources and skilled staff

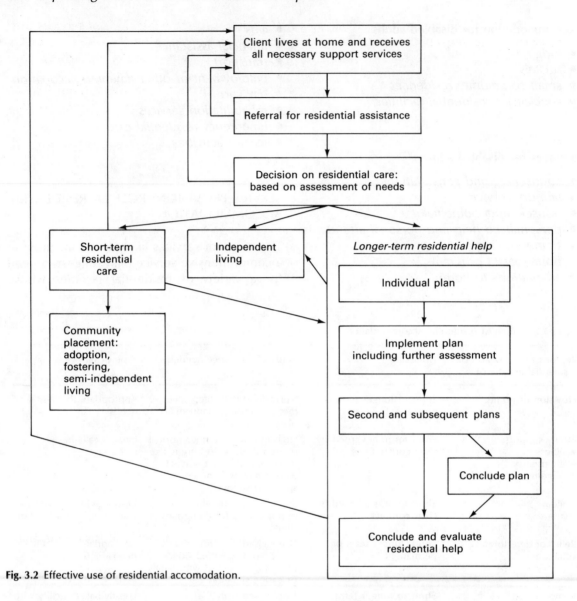

Fig. 3.2 Effective use of residential accomodation.

goals and ways of operating will differ according to:

- the nature and degree of assistance needed
- the reasons why accommodation is provided
- the time scale involved.

These issues are summarised in Table 3.1 and considered in greater detail in the next chapter.

A number of general principles should govern the use of residential facilities whatever their function:

- They should be made available as a result of clearly defined need; thus they should not be viewed as a place of last resort, to be used only when all other forms of help have been exhausted
- Clients should decide for themselves whether they wish to live in a particular residential setting
- Individuals should remain in a residence for as long as they are in need of the assistance and care it provides
- Provision of a place in a residence and its

likely duration should be the subject of a contract giving security to clients, but also, unless legal restrictions are imposed, allowing them to leave whenever they wish
- Residences for most disabled people should be as normal and homelike as possible; that is, they should:
  — be located within residential areas
  — look like the homes of other people
  — not provide for the total education, work, health and leisure needs of clients
- The pattern of daily life in a residence should be structured so that it develops personal skills and maximises maturation.

The general process governing the use of residential accommodation is suggested in Figure 3.2. Issues relating to referral and decision-making are discussed in the next chapter and help for individual clients is the subject of the second part of this book.

THE WAY FORWARD

This chapter has attempted to indicate future directions for the development of services for disabled people. While there is an urgent need to plan and make available comprehensive services, it should at the same time be recognised that this is likely to involve a considerable time scale. It does not, however, follow that organisations at present assisting disabled people can do nothing; they can, for example:

- begin to question the kinds of services they are at present providing
- clarify the value base from which they operate
- consider definitions of need they are using
- seek more effective ways of assisting clients.

For organisations providing residential services, their immediate goals are likely to include plans for:

- establishing intake systems
- developing smaller residences or group living arrangements within existing facilities
- developing individual plans
- reducing the degree of control staff have over clients
- increasing community involvement
- ensuring that helping approaches are consistent with the needs of clients and, where appropriate, those of families
- preparing statements relating to caring objectives and good practice, including:
  — the role of the facility within the overall service delivery system
  — client groups to be assisted
  — general goals sought for clients
  — client rights
  — relationships with families and their involvement in residential life
  — clear guidelines as to what constitutes good and bad care
  — client involvement in decision-making
  — a formal complaints system.

Need for intake systems
Admission to residential care: general
considerations
Characteristics of an intake system

4

Allocating residential services

Until quite recently, the need to regulate the use of residential accommodation through the operation of allocations systems went unrecognised. This was so because it was considered appropriate that disabled people problematic to themselves, their families or to society should be placed in institutions. Thus it was a matter of immediate admission or placement on a waiting list, and both the realities of limited resources and variations in need were factors not taken into account.

As a result of this approach, vacancies in residential facilities were allocated in whatever way seemed appropriate to those controlling them. This often resulted in:

- keeping strictly to the order of a waiting list regardless of need
- admitting people, however minimal their disabilities, to keep beds occupied
- exerting considerable pressure on senior residential staff to make places immediately available
- admitting people as favours for those involved with or having responsibility for disabled people.

The future use of all services for disabled people, and particularly residential accommodation, should be based on identified need and, where there are limitations in services, regulated by priority systems. To make services generally available, to provide them without either effective intake systems or clear evidence of need is unhelpful because to do so:

- represents an unnecessary use of scarce resources
- often means that those with greatest need do not receive assistance
- can be counter-productive to the real needs of clients and families
- prevents the development of more appropriate forms of assistance
- is contrary to the basic principles on which contemporary approaches to disabled people are based.

NEED FOR INTAKE SYSTEMS

Intake systems are:
> *formally agreed processes for co-ordinating requests for services and allocating vacancies.*

Once in use intake systems have considerable benefits for organisations, helpers, clients and their families in that they:

- assist in avoiding unnecessary and inappropriate use of resources and personnel
- reduce hasty and irrational decision-making
- provide opportunities for the participation of those likely to be affected by allocation decisions, particularly clients, families and direct care workers
- ensure that decisions relating to service provision are made by those competent to do so
- eliminate allocation of services based on hidden motives, undue pressure or preferencial consideration
- allocate services in terms of priority
- rationalise waiting lists and emergency admissions.

Since this book is intended for organisations providing residential accommodation, the remainder of this chapter considers the kind of intake process suited to residential services. The basic characteristics discussed, however, such as referral, decision-making, priority categories and waiting lists are relevant in the allocation of other services.

In general, before any service is provided, it is necessary to:

- collect sufficient information for rational decision-making
- undertake an appropriate assessment of need
- acknowledge which needs should be met
- appreciate the likely impact and consequences of services to be offered on all involved
- formulate a contract or understanding relating to services to be made available and obligations of those involved
- determine a time-scale for the provision of services.

ADMISSION TO RESIDENTIAL CARE: GENERAL CONSIDERATIONS

Before exploring the characteristics of an intake system for residential facilities, it is important to be aware of a number of general factors relating to the use of such accommodation. These factors concern:

> *Reasons for providing residential accommodation*
> *Counter-productive dimensions associated with residential life*
> *Time-scale of residential assistance*
> *Short-term residential care.*

Why provide residential accommodation?

Many of the reasons for providing residential accommodation have been indicated in the previous chapter. Among the more usual ones are:

- *To provide a home for clients.* Accommodation is often necessary because many disabled people are unable to provide for themselves. For such people residential care is likely to be long term
- *To support families.* Caring for some disabled children and adults is often physically and psychologically exhausting, and without some form of outside help, families often reach a point of breakdown. One most important way of providing support is by making regular periods of short-term

care available; this is often referred to as respite care. In addition to assisting families, such periods can be used to positively assist clients

- *To relieve deteriorating situations.* Even where families have successfully provided for their disabled members on a long-term basis, there is always a likelihood of change or deterioration. This is particularly the case where disabled adults are living with aged parents. In such situations the provision of residential accommodation may be necessary on a short- or longer-term basis.
- *Removal from an unsatisfactory situation.* Occasionally disabled people are found to be living in contexts where they are neglected or abused and so alternative accommodation on a short- or longer-term basis should be available
- *Assessment and investigation.* It is sometimes the case that it is impossible to make an appropriate assessment of both the needs of clients and difficulties encountered in caring for them while they are living with their families or in some other community setting. For these clients short-term residential assistance is appropriate
- *Development of client skills.* Because of the ways in which they are perceived and treated by their families when living at home, it is sometimes impossible for clients to develop sufficient skills to achieve appropriate levels of independence and social integration. Placement in a supportive and purposeful residential setting which is able to provide necessary skill development not only brings about growth, it demonstrates to those close to clients their potential for change.

Counter-productive nature of residential life

While it is clear that residential care has the potential to provide a great deal of assistance, those involved in decisions about its use for individual clients should be realistic about what can actually be attained. Accompanying many forms of residential care, in part

because of the legacy of past approaches, are several dimensions which are counter-productive to declared goals. While helpers will be aware of these limitations and be committed to eliminating them, they may be incapable of achieving much in the short term. It is important, therefore, before offering a place to a client, to balance what it is hoped to achieve against the realities of residential life.

Among some of the dimensions that should be considered are:

- *Abnormality of residential life.* Many facilities continue to operate with quite abnormal patterns of life and expectations of clients. As a result, some clients can actually be harmed by residential placement
- *Exposure to the stresses of residential life.* A number of factors make many residences stressful, particularly living in a group with similar disabilities and being isolated from mainstream society. These kinds of stresses are often far greater than those experienced by others living in their own homes and can be made worse by limitations in client coping skills
- *Multiple helpers.* It is an exceptional residence that operates over a period of time with a stable group of staff. Most residences experience continual movement of helpers which means that the extent of their commitment to and the quality of their relationships with clients cannot but be superficial
- *Loss of individuality.* While the expression of individuality is recognised as a basic need and entitlement in society, it is often the case that the size of some resident groups necessitates a pattern of life and routines which inhibit individual development
- *Stigma accompanying residential care.* Because of past beliefs, stigma continues to be attached to residential accommodation. Members of society believe that specialist residential resources are for abnormal people, and so both clients and those close to them become negatively regarded.

Clients themselves are often conscious of these stigmatising consequences which contribute to their devalued self-identity.

Time-scale of residential assistance

As a result of the past function of residential facilities, admission usually meant long-term care. It was rare for clients to move from a residence to the community and so the need for varying lengths of stay was not recognised.

Today, as the above discussion on reasons for providing residential accommodation suggests, the time scale should be related to client need and so may range from overnight to longer-term care. It is thus the case that it will be unrelated to the professional needs of staff or the rules and traditions of a residence.

Providing assistance that reflects client need in terms of length of stay may involve:

- designating a specific number of places for short-term as against longer-term assistance
- setting up specialist residences for differing lengths of stay
- changing approaches to care to accommodate a continual movement of clients
- changing funding structures.

Short-term residential care

Short-term care is likely to increase once it is recognised that residential accommodation has an important part to play in supporting family life. Among the specific areas of need short-term care can meet are:

- providing relief for parents and others caring for disabled people where the task is physically or psychologically exhausting
- providing opportunities for clients to have holidays in situations where their specialised needs can be met
- relief for full-time carers to enable them to do things they otherwise could not do
- crisis situations such as family breakdown or illness in carers.

Once families know of and can come to rely on short-term care, the strain of caring is reduced and any sense of burden is felt to be less immense.

In establishing a system of short-term care, it is necessary to:

- determine criteria for offering short-term placements
- identify in what residences or other caring settings short-term accommodation is to be made available, and make the number of available places known
- devise an administrative system which will co-ordinate and plan intake
- ensure that an understanding or contract exists about the return of clients to their usual place of residence.

CHARACTERISTICS OF AN INTAKE SYSTEM

An intake system governing one or more residential facilities will include details of:

> *Clients to be assisted and services offered*
> *A point of contact for referral*
> *A decision-making process*
> *The use of waiting lists*
> *Emergency placement*
> *Pre-placement planning*
> *Client reception.*

The various stages from referral for residential assistance to reception in a residence are set out in Figure 4.1.

Clients to be assisted and services offered

It is necessary for each residence to operate with a clear understanding about the clients it seeks to assist. Such an understanding will follow from the role allocated to and accepted by a facility within a comprehensive service plan. Among the reasons why such a statement should exist and be used to regulate intake are that:

- it is unfair to individual clients to admit them to residences which assist groups, either in age, personal characteristics or disability, that are markedly different from them

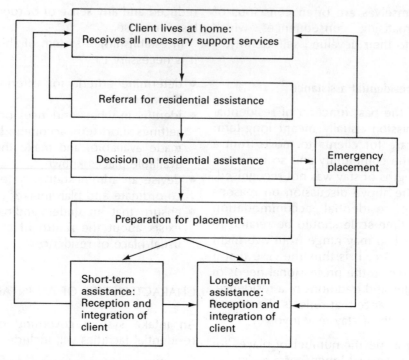

Fig. 4.1 Process of referral, decision-making and reception.

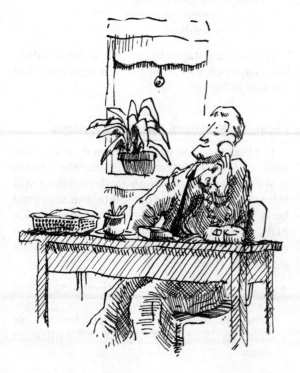

- staff have difficulty in providing the right kind of assistance where clients and their needs vary a great deal.

A point of contact for referral

Requests for residential accommodation are made by many people, for example, clients themselves, their families and friends, neighbours and professional workers. In order to deal effectively with such requests, it is necessary for an organisation, or a group of organisations operating together, to make available a single point of referral, be it an individual or team of workers, to provide advice or to enable the first steps in requesting placement to be taken.

A point of referral is an important and essential screening step. In the hands of capable workers it can be of help to the person making the enquiry and save considerable time and effort for those involved at the

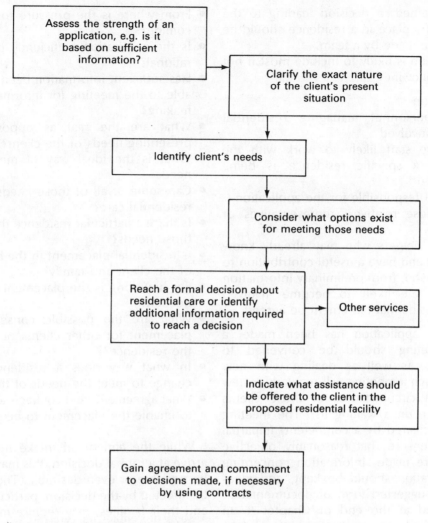

Fig. 4.2 Responding to requests for residential assistance.

decision-making stage. Where a request for residential assistance is clearly inappropriate, practical advice can be given on other services that may be more helpful. Whatever advice is offered at this preliminary stage, those making the initial approach on behalf of a client should be entitled to proceed with a formal application where they consider it essential.

Referral discussions will focus upon:

- the needs and presenting problems of clients
- reasons for referral and help sought

- what placement in a residential facility might achieve
- the likelihood of a vacancy being available
- the possible length of any waiting period
- further steps to be taken including the collection of information for an intake meeting.

A decision-making process

Because of its importance in the allocation of limited resources and its significance for the client concerned, a decision leading to the provision of a place in a residence should be a formal one made by a team.

Such a team is likely to include most if not all of the following:

- chairperson
- senior personnel managing residential facilities involved
- direct-care staff likely to work with the client if a specific residence is being considered
- individual responsible for the application
- client, close relatives, representatives or advocates
- specialist helpers who may already know the client and have a useful contribution to make or who, from preliminary information available, are likely to become involved should residential placement be agreed.

Once an application has been made, a formal meeting should be convened to consider it. As well as dealing with new requests, such a meeting will regularly review the present circumstances of those clients who may be on a waiting list. The meeting should be chaired by a competent, impartial person to ensure that reasonably objective decisions are made. Information concerning each application should be kept, and ideas towards a suggested form of documentation are included at the end of Chapter 9. In responding˙ to an application, an intake meeting is likely to follow a series of steps such as those outlined Figure 4.2.

There are many important questions an intake meeting should consider. In situations where clients and their families have receiving some form of help, most answers may already be known. Among such questions are:

- From where is the pressure for placement coming?
- Is the application sufficiently detailed and rational?
- Has sufficient information been made available to the meeting for informed decision-making?
- What are the real as opposed to the presenting needs of the client?
- What is the ideal way of meeting those needs?
- Can some or all of those needs be met by residential care?
- Is there a particular residence that can meet those needs?
- Is residential placement in the best interest of the client and family?
- For how long is the placement likely to be needed?
- What are the possible consequences of placement for other clients or for staff in the residence?
- In what way does a residence need to change to meet the needs of the client?
- What agreements and contracts are necessary to enable the placement to be successful?

While the aim of an intake meeting is to arrive at a formal decision, this may not always be possible or even desirable. Those likely to be affected by the decision, particularly clients and their families, may require more time to consider the consequences of admission or to explore alternatives in greater depth. In any event, they will probably want to visit the proposed establishment before making up their minds. The final decision, therefore, may need to be made at a later meeting or delegated to the chairperson to take at the appropriate time.

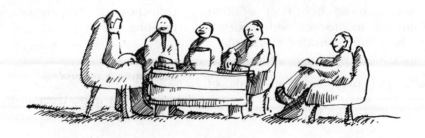

Where a request for residential care is refused, such a decision should not be communicated in any final or arbitrary way. The reasons should be made known to all concerned, and those making the original application should feel free to re-apply whenever they consider it necessary.

Once a decision has been made and a place becomes available, a formal and fully documented understanding or contract, involving all those who will have responsibilities in relation to the client, should be drawn up. This contract should include:

- a statement about the help the residential facility will provide
- the responsibilities of staff
- the responsibilities of parents or relatives, particularly in terms of continued contact and involvement
- the responsibilities of the client
- the length of placement, including any trial period
- criteria for prematurely ending or extending placement.

Waiting lists

Since the number of available places in residential accommodation will often be limited, it will be necessary to maintain waiting lists. In order to avoid large and meaningless lists which can have unhelpful consequences for clients and for organisations assisting them, their use should be governed by the following factors:

- names of clients will be added only as a result of a decision made at an intake meeting
- the circumstances of each client on a waiting list will be reviewed at regular intervals
- the ordering of a list will be based on agreed criteria for determining priority
- information should be given to clients and their families about the priority system in use, their position on the waiting list and the likely time period before placement is possible.

Table 4.1 Priority categories for residential services

Category 1	Situations where, because of a serious threat to a client's well being or that of others, there is an urgent need for residential accommodation.
Category 2	Situations that will, without residential assistance, deteriorate so that they fall into Category 1.
Category 3	Situations that will get worse if residential assistance is not provided.
Category 4	Situations where the client will benefit from residential assistance.
Category 5	Situations where there is no real need for residential assistance or where it is unlikely to bring about any significant benefit.

Devising priority systems is far from easy and there is at present no simple way of identifying those clients whose needs for residential assistance are greatest. In general, in whatever way a waiting list is ordered, it should range from clients who have needs suggesting admission at the earliest possible moment to those who will not be adversely affected by remaining where they are. The categories in Table 4.1 may assist some organisations in establishing their own priority system.

A waiting list should be reviewed regularly, particularly when the names of more clients are added to it. The likely outcome of such reviews will be that those whose needs are not urgent in comparison with others are unlikely ever to be offered placement. Where this is so, it should be made known to all concerned and more appropriate services made available.

Emergency placement

While there will always be a need for emergency placements, they can cause immense problems and so should not be viewed as necessary or desirable. They can, for example:

- be based on totally inadequate information
- create in staff a sense of panic
- make nonsense of waiting lists
- be engineered to obtain placement

- render preparation of clients almost impossible
- be an inappropriate way of dealing with a crisis and so make matters worse.

An emergency placement should be made only when the circumstances of a client suggest it to be essential, that is where:

- the client is abused in a way that endangers his or her life, is cruelly treated or is deprived of certain essential necessities such as food, clothing, and shelter
- other people living with the client are being abused by the client
- those who have provided essential care are no longer available.

A formal procedure should be adopted for emergency admissions which will include:

- an understanding that an admission will be for a limited period of time, and will be terminated if it is found to have been unnecessary or if others on a waiting list have greater priority
- a condition that placement will end when the circumstances creating the emergency no longer exist
- a requirement that, shortly after admission, full information be provided about the client and the situation giving rise to the emergency.

Despite difficulties associated with emergency admissions, they serve the purpose of relieving very stressful situations and provide real help to clients and their families. But they should be made only when genuine vacancies exists. The beds of clients who happen to be away should never be used for emergencies.

Pre-placement planning

Moving from home or some other living situation to a residential setting is likely to be a major event in the lives of many clients. It is important to prepare them for it, both to minimise the effects of a potentially disturbing experience and to create positive feelings.

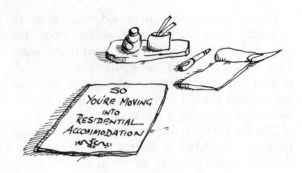

Among the aspects of pre-placement planning may be:

Acquainting clients with the decision if they have not helped to make it.
Exclusion of clients from the decision-making process should be a rare occurrence. Where it has been unavoidable, the reasons why residential care is thought to be desirable should be explained to them. If clients or those close to them object, placement should not proceed.

Providing clients and their families with information about the proposed residence.
This is best done in discussion and by making available a booklet containing relevant information. Some of the topics for inclusion in such a booklet may be:

- description and illustrations of the residence
- its formal objectives
- client involvement in daily life
- services available and help that can be expected from staff
- limitations on length of stay
- expectations about family involvement
- financial aspects
- support services
- the pattern of daily life, programs and activities
- community involvement
- details of what personal possessions clients should bring.

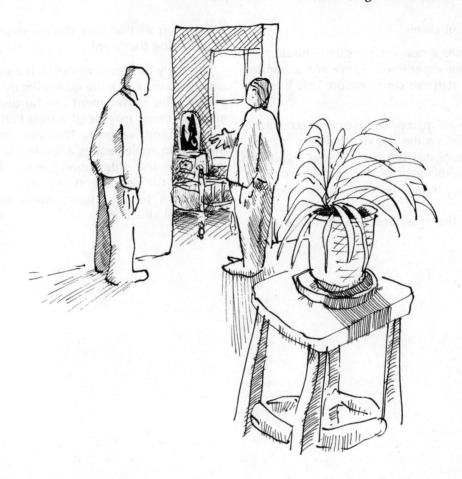

Visiting the client at home.

A visit to a client at home is best undertaken by a helper who is likely to become significant following placement. Seeing clients at home provides helpers with a broader understanding of them and is an initial step in establishing positive relationships. At the same time, such visits enable clients and their families to ask questions about life in the residential facility in a setting where they do not feel disadvantaged.

Client visiting the residence.

Where clients or their families have any doubts about accepting a placement, a visit can help them make up their minds.

It will also enable the client to become familiar with the residence and meet other residents and staff.

Overnight stay.

An overnight stay makes it possible for clients to experience something of the pattern of life of a residence, and gives staff and other residents the chance to get to know clients before they move in.

Arranging the day and time for placement.

The day and time chosen should be convenient for all involved, particularly for the client and any helpers and residents who may be involved in the reception process.

Reception of clients

Moving into a new environment should be a pleasurable experience. There are a number of things staff can do to ensure that it is; for example:

- identify an appropriate person to accompany the client on the day of admission
- make sure that the client brings significant personal belongings, for example, clothes, photos, books, electrical appliances, toys, pets
- ensure that reception is relaxed and avoids experiences that have the consequences of devaluing the client.

The early days and weeks in the new living situation are likely to be quite difficult for many clients. The environment can be disorienting and the client may need sympathetic understanding and support. The time and effort involved in implementing a sensitively prepared reception and integration period helps to eliminate the depression and sense of loneliness often felt by clients when moving to residential situations.

PART | **TWO**

Meeting individual need

Contemporary approaches emphasise the capacity of disabled people to develop and become mature, and the responsibility of those assisting them to provide appropriate personalised help to make this possible. Nowhere is help of this kind more necessary than in the residential context. An analysis of the operation of many residences suggests the help clients have available to them to be limited by inadequate conceptions of need and practical and personalised ways providing assistance. It is not enough now to seek a general improvement in their pattern of life, it is necessary to develop individualised ways of enabling them to become as independent and as responsible for themselves as they are able, to live normal lives and to become integrated into mainstream society.

The five chapters that follow focus on ways of achieving these goals by means of an individual orientation. Chapter 5 discusses a systematic way of individualising help, that is, individual planning. Chapter 6 looks at client need and ways in which it can be assessed, and provides an example of the kind of check-list that can be used when assessing some of the more important personal and social skills. Chapter 7 discusses how programming can enhance skill development for those clients who experience difficulty in learning, and Chapter 8 describes some of the teaching strategies that can be used in programming. Finally, Chapter 9 considers client records and the importance of appropriate documentation in the helping process.

5

A client-centred focus: individual planning

In the past, residential care for disabled people was justified on the grounds that, in being a burden to families and a nuisance to the wider society, special accommodation was necessary for their isolation and containment. As a consequence, the operational philosophies of most residential settings excluded a client-centred focus and conceptions of individualised need. Following admission, new inmates were simply absorbed into the institutional regime and expected to conform regardless of their own needs and wishes or the extent to which the pattern of life was of benefit to them. Even in the exceptional residence where helpers attempted to provide more than containment, efforts were rarely based on any meaningful understanding of client need.

If residential services are to operate in ways that reflect contemporary beliefs about disabled people, it is essential that patterns of life and forms of help are consistent with client need. One of the major ways in which this can be achieved is through the development of plans for clients which identify need and detail appropriate helping responses.

Various organisations and professional groups workings with disabled people use different terms for such plans. These include:

- case plans
- individual program plans
- individual treatment plans
- individual development plans

- individual habilitation plans
- individual life plans.

While each term refers to a similar process, the one used in this book is *individual plan*, not so much because it more accurately defines such a plan but because it avoids conceptual limitations associated with the others.

An individual plan can be defined as:

> *a systematic process of intervention which aims at identifying and meeting the needs of a client.*

At some stage in a disabled person's stay in residential accommodation, irrespective of age or disability, such a plan will be essential if needs are to be met.

Individual plans can achieve a great deal for clients; for example, they:

- enable a holistic understanding to be attained, that is, one that comprehends their needs in relation to their total life situation
- enable needs to be identified and the necessary services and helping approaches to be made available
- ensure that the efforts of helpers assisting clients are co-ordinated, rational and consistent
- prevent clients being forgotten and their needs overlooked.

Since the idea of individual planning may be quite new to many organisations working with disabled people, this chapter aims primarily at acquainting helpers with the processes involved in developing and using such plans. The final section puts forward some practical suggestions for their introduction to residential settings.

INDIVIDUAL PLANS FOR ALL CLIENTS?

While the idea of individual planning represents a significant development in improving assistance to disabled people, it is important to be aware that there is something artificial about such a process. Few other members of society have their lives systematically shaped and organised, and so it is an approach to help that should only be used when it is of real benefit to clients. At some point in time, therefore, a decision may have to be made for most clients about discontinuing individual planning. This is an issue considered later in the chapter.

A TEAMWORK AND INTERDISCIPLINARY APPROACH

Growth in the helping professions has resulted in a number of groups becoming involved in residential services for disabled people, and most organisations today will be employing helpers from a variety of disciplines. Despite their expertise, the success they have had in assisting clients has been quite limited. This has been so for a number of reasons. First, as has already been suggested, the custodial role of the institution tended to have a neutralising effect on efforts to help. Second, no integrated notions of helping were ever established. Third, trained helpers tended to operate in isolation from one another and often with competing conceptions of client need. Fourth, direct care staff were viewed as being incapable of acting in other than custodial roles, and so were excluded from efforts to assist clients in positive ways. Finally, clients and their families were expected to be passive recipients of expert help and denied information about themselves and involvement in decision making.

Problems and defects such as these can be overcome by developing individual plans within a teamwork and interdisciplinary approach, that is, one that combines the insights and helping skills of a range of people to arrive at a comprehensive understanding of client need and the appropriate helping resources to meet it. A teamwork and interdisciplinary approach requires from all involved an orientation which:

- acknowledges that an understanding of the needs of most clients can be attained only through the combined efforts of a group of people contributing differing kinds of expertise

- seeks to make decisions by consensus rather than on the basis of seniority or assumed expertise
- makes decisions only in relation to accurate information, and not on conjecture or hypothesis
- encourages the sharing of information as plans are developed, implemented and reviewed
- provides on-going support to other members of the team as they implement their part of the plan
- accepts that once plans have been formulated and agreed they are binding on members.

The benefits of a teamwork and interdisciplinary approach for clients are obvious. Such an approach also has numerous benefits for helpers, particularly in broadening outlooks, knowledge and understandings, and in extending skills.

RESPONSIBILITIES OF PLANNING TEAMS

Since the needs of individual clients are so varied, the composition of teams responsible for preparing individual plans will differ. In general, membership of a planning team will be limited to those helpers who are assisting a client. Since size is an important factor in the success of planning teams, some workers may need to be represented by others. Among the disciplines likely to be involved are:

- residential staff working directly with clients
- medical practitioners
- nurses
- teachers
- psychologists
- social workers
- occupational therapists
- psysiotherapists
- speech pathologists.

Preparing individual plans should not be seen as something done to or on behalf of clients by staff, but should, wherever possible, be a joint enterprise involving helpers, clients, their families and representatives. Thus a planning team is likely to include the client and others close to him/her, be they family members, personal friends or those in an advocate role.

The broad task of a team will be to prepare, implement and review individual plans by:

- obtaining and evaluating information concerning client need
- agreeing on needs to be met
- placing those needs in some order of priority
- identifying appropriate helping contexts and approaches
- nominating people to carry out specific tasks in relation to identified needs.

Since planning teams are of considerable importance to the welfare of clients, they should be accorded due recognition and given sufficient power to allocate resources and assign work tasks.

It is likely that there will be areas of need that cannot be met by the members of a planning team, and these may include health, education and housing needs. A team should, therefore, through its co-ordinator, seek to involve others in the planning process by inviting them to attend appropriate meetings or through discussion with the co-ordinator.

CO-ORDINATING PLANS

It is essential that individual workers assume responsibility for co-ordinating client plans. This responsibility can be assigned in one of two ways:

- appointing one or more persons to act as *plan co-ordinators* for a residence, so having responsibility for the plans of many clients
- designating individuals to act as *key workers* for specific clients and assigning

them responsibility for co-ordinating plans. Key workers should be individuals who are close and significant to clients and who are involved in assisting them. It may be possible for some clients or relatives to act on their own behalf in this role.

In whatever way the role of co-ordinator is assigned, among the responsibilities of the person involved will be to ensure that:

- planning and review meetings are held
- satisfactory plans are prepared
- those agreeing to assist clients and their families do so
- those assisting clients communicate and co-operate on an ongoing basis
- needs which cannot be met by members of planning teams or others represented by them are met in some other way
- appropriate records are kept.

CONTENT OF PLANS

The broad and varying needs of clients make it impossible to provide a comprehensive statement about what should be included in individual plans. Some of the important areas of need will be:

- health
- family
- education
- mobility and transport
- communication
- vocation and work
- leisure
- self-help
- personal development and identity
- daily living
- community integration.

This list is expanded in the next chapter specifically to highlight areas where assessment may be necessary.

DEVELOPING AND REVIEWING PLANS

Figure 5.1 summarises the kind of process that

is involved in developing and reviewing individual plans. Its various aspects are discussed below and in later chapters.

First plan

The initial plan should normally be prepared in the first month. While considerable information may already exist, the first plan is likely to be a tentative one because, not only will specific forms of assessment need to be carried out which may render information obtained before admission somewhat irrelevant, but the client may respond in unexpected ways in the new environment making necessary quite new approaches.

However tentative the initial plan, it should attempt to detail:

- total needs of a client, irrespective of whether they can be met
- forms of assessment that should be undertaken
- needs that can be met while the client is living in residential accommodation
- the ordering of those needs in terms of importance to the client
- ways in which they can be met
- the actual needs to be responded to
- responsibilities of the various agencies and workers involved
- what contracts should be made
- the date for a formal review of the plan.

Second plan

At an agreed time following the preparation of the first plan, and probably between eight and sixteen weeks, a formal review should be undertaken by a planning team with the aim of drawing up a new plan.

The specific tasks of such a review will be to:

- consider the extent to which needs detailed in the first plan are being met
- enable the client to review what has been happening
- evaluate the client's response to helping approaches

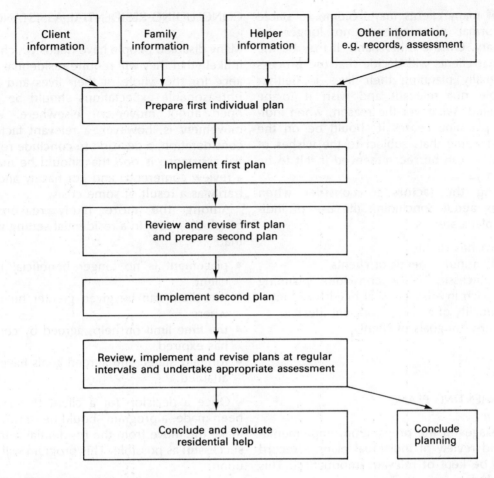

Fig. 5.1 Developing and reviewing plans.

- enable staff to comprehend what is happening with the client
- provide practical suggestions for responding to specific needs
- oblige staff to account for the nature and quality of their work with the client
- detail and prioritise new needs
- consider approaches necessary for meeting these needs
- review contracts made when the first plan was prepared.

At the conclusion of a formal review the co-ordinator, or key worker, should ensure that a revised individual plan is drawn up and made available. This plan will include:

- a summary of the points discussed

- a statement of new goals
- details as to how these goals are to be pursued
- details of new contracts that need to be made.

Third and subsequent plans

At regular intervals of between six and nine months, or more frequently if it appears necessary, further conferences should be held to review individual plans. The process followed will be similar to that outlined above.

Concluding planning

It is probable that at some point in time the

lives of many clients may become so stable that formal planning will no longer be necessary. On the other hand, it may be the case that clients will decide that the process of formally planning their lives is neither desirable nor relevant and wish it to be terminated. Whatever the reason, when individual planning ceases it should be on the understanding that, subject to the wishes of a client, it can be recommenced if felt to be necessary.

Among the factors to consider when thinking about concluding the use of individual plans are:

- the wishes clients
- the continuing needs of clients
- the necessity of a conscious planning approach in ensuring that needs are met
- the quality of a client's present lifestyle
- longer-term goals of clients.

DOCUMENTING PLANS

At all stages in the preparation, implementation and review of individual plans a record should be kept of relevant information. This will include:

- information obtained for the purpose of identifying need, including personal history and assessment
- a formal and updated statement of needs
- details of specific needs which a team will attempt to meet
- details of helping responses
- organisations and personnel who have accepted responsibility for meeting specified needs
- ongoing information relating to a client's changing lifestyle
- evaluation of the help that has been provided.

The type of form on which suitable information can be recorded is outlined in Chapter 9.

CONCLUDING RESIDENTIAL ASSISTANCE

Many disabled people have needs which make it likely that they will require residential assistance for the whole of their lives and so no unreasonable expectations should be developed about movement elsewhere. Where movement is, however, a relevant factor for consideration, a decision to conclude residential assistance is one that should be made at a review conference and not hastily and arbitrarily as a result of some crisis.

Among the more likely reasons for concluding care in a residential setting will be that:

- placement is no longer beneficial to the client
- the client can be given greater help elsewhere
- the time limit on help, agreed by contract, has expired
- formally stated and agreed goals have been attained.

Once a decision for a client to leave has been made, a program should be drawn up to make the move from the residential setting as successful as possible. This program will focus upon:

- the ways in which the client and other may need to be prepared
- action necessary to prepare any new living environment
- the extent of any necessary support, including day services
- identifying the most appropriate time for the move.

The needs of clients will be uppermost when such plans are being devised, and residential staff should accept that their obligations may not necessarily end once clients have left a residence. Successes achieved by clients can be undermined by inadequate preparation programs or through failure to provide sufficient on-going services and support both to clients and others close to them in their new living environment.

INTRODUCING THE PLANNING PROCESS

As indicated earlier in this chapter, some organisations assisting disabled people may be unfamiliar with individual plans. Since these plans are now seen as the basis for identifying and meeting client need, it is essential that steps are taken to introduce them. How this is achieved will vary from organisation to organisation. For the majority, the most effective way will be to start with one client, and then extend the process to others, for example:

Step 1   Discuss with staff and clients the idea of individual plans, and the concepts on which they are based, including planning, reviewing, recording.

Step 2   Identify a particular client for whom an individual plan is necessary and obtain his or her agreement to the preparation of a plan.

Step 3   Arrange a meeting and invite to it all those involved with the client, including the client, close relatives and the client's representative.

Step 4   Focus the meeting on identifying needs and deciding forms of help. Operate with a concept of need which is limited to the forms of assistance that realistically can be offered. Record a plan of action following the meeting and the responsibilities of those involved.

Step 5   Implement the plan.

Step 6   After an agreed period of time, meet again to review what has happened and to prepare a revised plan.

As staff become familiar with such a process, develop the ability to work together in planning meetings and can put into practice what has been agreed, individual planning can be extended to other clients, involve other helpers, be based on wider definitions of need and use a greater variety of helping approaches.

6

Identifying and assessing need

The previous chapter presented an overview of individual planning, and this present one explores the first stage in the planning process, that is, identifying and assessing need.

The idea of assessment has been central to the functioning of the helping professions almost since their inception, and today a number of forms of assessment are used with disabled people. An analysis of many of them, however, suggests that while they at first appear oriented to identifying client need, they do, in fact, serve to attain quite different goals. Many measures of assessment, for example, in having been developed in relation to the beliefs of particular professional groups, assert views of clients which have the function of reinforcing those beliefs. In the hands of some groups, assessment has been refined to the point where it is understood only by those using it, so justifying the exclusion of others from the assessment process. At the extreme, some forms of assessment are desired as ends in themselves, and are of little relevance to clients, their families and direct care workers.

If assessment is to provide useful information on which helping approaches can be based, those assisting disabled people should appreciate that:

- client agreement to and active involvement in assessment is essential
- assessment is of value only if it results in

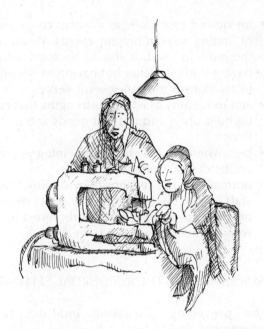

the identification of needs which, in relation to individual clients, can and should be met

- all forms of assessment are based on certain beliefs, such as those, for example, of the social worker interviewing parents about the desirability of residential care for their child to those implicit in many standardised tests
- each form of assessment, because of limitations in orientation and assessment techniques, provides only a partial understanding of need
- information gained by assessment is often shaped by factors in the client's immediate environment. In residential situations, for example, relationships with others or stresses arising from daily life can influence outcomes.

WHAT IS ASSESSMENT?

Assessment can be understood as:

the process by which information relating to clients is collected, organised and interpreted so that informed decisions about needs and how they can be responded to can be made.

Assessment provides clients, families and those assisting them with practical information concerning:

- personal and interpersonal functioning
- past and present factors affecting a client's life experiences
- aspects of life clients and others consider to be important.

There are a number of forms of assessment that are useful in assisting disabled people and each serves a different purpose and obtains specific kinds of information. Among them are:

- interviewing: finding out, as a result of discussion with clients, close relatives and other significant people, what are viewed as the more important needs
- reviewing personal history and records: this enables helpers to identify what needs have been suggested in the past and others that may be implied
- observation: both structured and unstructured observations can be undertaken in a variety of settings to identify what the needs of clients appear to be
- testing: using checklists, standardised tests, and questionnaires to identify need.

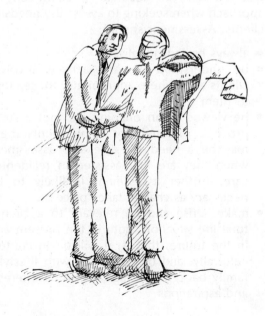

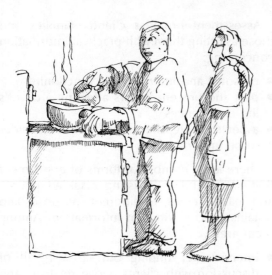

Before any form of assessment is used it is important to clarify reasons for its use and the kinds of information it is hoped can be obtained. It is important also, after undertaking assessment, to review the assessment process, together with information obtained, to identify factors that may have affected outcomes. Finally, if a detailed and holistic understanding of a client is sought, it is necessary to combine a number of forms of assessment.

The following principles suggest a framework which can lead to a client-centred approach when seeking to assess the needs of clients. Assessment should:

- always be individualised
- be understood by, and actively involve, clients and, where appropriate, those close to them
- be viewed as an ongoing and not a static process. Although for some clients there may be a need for extensive assessment when they are first assisted in residential care, further assessment is likely to be necessary as change takes place
- make sense and be relevant to a client's total life situation, both in the present and in the future, that is, it will be in context culturally, and be consistent with lifestyle, family background, age, personal interests and aspirations

- be viewed essentially as a means to an end, of finding ways of helping clients. Whatever the method used, it should be seen not as having intrinsic value but having worth only in relation to the purposes it serves
- aim to identify assets and strengths that can be built upon and not just needs and problems
- be, wherever possible, an integral and unobstrusive aspect of daily life
- normally be the responsibility of direct care staff. Consultants and advisers should become involved only where direct care workers need their assistance.

ASSESSMENT IN THE RESIDENTIAL SETTING

The preceding discussion indicates that assessment should be:

- individualised and related to the needs of the client
- in context
- oriented to obtaining information on which positive programs of action can be based.

Deciding on appropriate forms of assessment for individual clients in residential settings should be the responsibility of planning teams. Factors influencing decisions will include:

- the nature and quality of information already available. Considerable information will have been obtained before a client

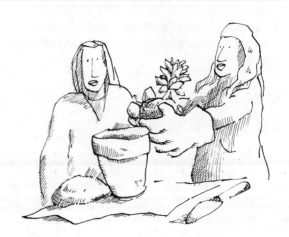

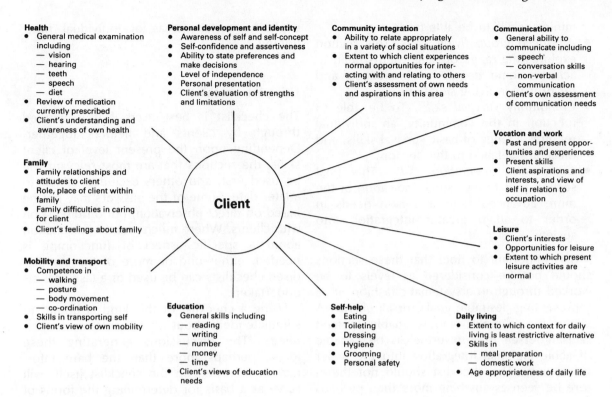

Health
- General medical examination including
  - vision
  - hearing
  - teeth
  - speech
  - diet
- Review of medication currently prescribed
- Client's understanding and awareness of own health

Family
- Family relationships and attitudes to client
- Role, place of client within family
- Family difficulties in caring for client
- Client's feelings about family

Mobility and transport
- Competence in
  - walking
  - posture
  - body movement
  - co-ordination
- Skills in transporting self
- Client's view of own mobility

Personal development and identity
- Awareness of self and self-concept
- Self-confidence and assertiveness
- Ability to state preferences and make decisions
- Level of independence
- Personal presentation
- Client's evaluation of strengths and limitations

Education
- General skills including
  - reading
  - writing
  - number
  - money
  - time
- Client's views of education needs

Community integration
- Ability to relate appropriately in a variety of social situations
- Extent to which client experiences normal opportunities for interacting with and relating to others
- Client's assessment of own needs and aspirations in this area

Self-help
- Eating
- Toileting
- Dressing
- Hygiene
- Grooming
- Personal safety

Communication
- General ability to communicate including
  - speech
  - conversation skills
  - non-verbal communication
- Client's own assessment of communication needs

Vocation and work
- Past and present opportunities and experiences
- Present skills
- Client aspirations and interests, and view of self in relation to occupation

Leisure
- Client's interests
- Opportunities for leisure
- Extent to which present leisure activities are normal

Daily living
- Extent to which context for daily living is least restrictive alternative
- Skills in
  - meal preparation
  - domestic work
- Age appropriateness of daily life

Client

Fig. 6.1 Aspects of life that may require assessment.

moved into a residence, and a review of it will give some indication of gaps
- reasons for the provision of residential assistance
- what clients identify as their major areas of need
- present skills of clients
- what appear to be the more obvious or presenting needs.

Figure 6.1 is an elaboration of the list in the previous chapter. It details areas of a client's life that may require assessment. It should be noted that what has been included in this chart is far from comprehensive. Selection of areas reflects the belief that help given to clients in residential contexts should focus on providing a satisfactory lifestyle that leads to greater competence and independence in everyday aspects of life and to greater community integration.

A RESIDENTIAL CHECKLIST

The checklist at the end of this chapter has been developed from some of the areas of need detailed in Figure 6.1. It attempts to set out those aspects of client functioning that are an appropriate focus for the helping approaches of staff in residential facilities. It is based on an awareness that in order to function effectively clients will need to possess a wide range of skills, from those in basic self care to those which enhance integration into community life. The checklist is divided into five sections:

- *Self-help skills.* This section looks at the skills a person requires to be able to function with some degree of independence in the most basic areas of life.
- *Basic group living skills.* In the residential situation disabled people live in a group context and this section focuses upon the

minimal skills to be able to do so.

- *Advanced group living skills.* This section explores the range of skills clients need to achieve some degree of interaction and reciprocity in living situations.
- *Community survival skills.* To be able to function in the community, an individual requires a range of basic survival skills, and these are detailed in this section.
- *Community integration skills.* This final section tries to give some indication of the more advanced skills a person needs in order to attain greater integration into society.

It is important to note that these sections should not be considered as levels to be worked through in a systematic fashion or as representing desirable goals for all clients. A client, for example, who is unable to feed himself/herself may nevertheless be capable of achieving total integration into the wider community. The checklist should not therefore be seen as anything more than perhaps a useful but also quite limited device for exploring certain areas of individual functioning.

Using the checklist

The checklist is best used if it is worked through by clients and helpers together. Depending upon the present level of client skills, the sections that are most relevant will be used first, and others excluded or left to a later date. Some of the answers may not be based on direct observation, but on discussion with clients. Where much greater information about a specific aspect of functioning is needed, either one or more of the standardised checklists can be used or a task analysis undertaken.

Using a checklist of this kind is bound to stimulate ideas about what clients see as their needs. The discussions generating these ideas, perhaps more than the bare information recorded on the checklist itself, will serve as a basis for determining the forms of help to be made available.

CLIENT SKILLS: A RESIDENTIAL CHECKLIST

Self-help skills

	Can do without assistance	Can do with assistance	Cannot do
Eating:			
• feeds self			
Toileting:			
• aware of requiring toilet			
• uses toilet by self			
Clothing:			
• dresses and undresses self — simple clothing			
Grooming and hygiene:			
• takes bath/shower when necessary			
• washes hands/face when necessary			
• cleans teeth			

Basic group living skills

	Can do without assistance	Can do with assistance	Cannot do
Eating:			
• shares food with others			
• uses cutlery appropriately			
• serves self with reasonable quantities of food and drink			
• eats with mouth closed, no spilling			
• prepares simple drinks and snacks			
Toileting:			
• flushes and leaves toilet clean			
• adjusts clothing			
• washes hands			
• recognises need for privacy			
Clothing:			
• fastens buttons, zips, laces			
• selects appropriate clothing for the day ..			
• stores clothing in cupboard/drawers			
• knows when clothes need washing or mending			
Grooming and hygiene:			
• keeps hair tidy			
• washes hair as necessary			
• cuts nails as necessary			
• shaves as necessary			
• uses tissues or handkerchieves appropriately			
• changes soiled clothing as necessary			
Decision-making:			
• participates in basic decision-making processes, e.g. daily routine, leisure and outings			

Advanced group living skills

	Can do without assistance	Can do with assistance	Cannot do
Personal safety:			
• shows awareness of hazards and dangers in home environment, e.g. poisons			
• exercises caution, e.g. hot objects, cigarettes			
• knows how to obtain help in emergency, e.g. use of phone			
• protects self appropriately			
Communication:			
• makes self known to others			
• holds basic conversation			
• communicates needs			
First aid/health:			
• indicates when sick			
• seeks help in emergency			
• treats simple injuries			
• knows and administers own medication ..			
Grooming and hygiene:			
• copes with menstruation appropriately			
Interactions with others:			
• able to say please and thank you			
• greets others appropriately			
• shows affection in appropriate way			
• assists others			
• respects privacy			
• controls behaviour			
• shares or lends with discretion			
• values the property of others			
• some awareness of feelings of others			

	Can do without assistance	Can do with assistance	Cannot do
Meal preparation:			
• stores, refrigerates, freezes food appropriately			
• assembles equipment, prepares ingredients			
• prepares and cooks simple meals			
• knows how to use domestic equipment, e.g.			
hot plate			
oven			
refrigerator			
toaster			
electric frypan			
kettle/jug			
dishwasher			
Domestic work			
• participates in and shares chores			
• sets table			
• washes up after meals			
• cleans and tidies living area			
• makes bed			
• washes and dries clothes			
• knows how to use:			
washing machine			
iron			
clothes dryer			
vacuum cleaner			
broom and mop			
• removes rubbish			
• maintains garden			

	Can do without assistance	Can do with assistance	Cannot do
Clothing:			
• dresses self completely			
• irons simple articles			
• keeps shoes in good condition and repair ...			
Leisure:			
• has hobbies and interests			
• participates in organised activities			
Time:			
• knows days of the week			
• tells time			
• knows times of basic activities and routines			
Personal knowledge:			
• knows own name, age, address			
Telephone:			
• answers home phone			
• dials number if written down			
• knows own phone number			

Community survival skills

	Can do without assistance	Can do with assistance	Cannot do
Movement in local community:			
• locates own house and street			
• uses key to front door			
• finds way around neighbourhood			
• locates shops and other places of importance, e.g. bank, post office, etc.			

	Can do without assistance	Can do with assistance	Cannot do
Public transport:			
• recognises bus, taxi stop and railway stations			
• gets on and off transport appropriately ...			
• pays fare and states destination			
• behaves appropriately on public transport ...			
Personal safety:			
• observes safety rules for crossing roads ..			
• understands traffic lights			
• understands pedestrian signs			
Communication:			
• makes own address or phone number known to others			
• asks for help or direction			
• uses public phone			
• names key workers, family address, phone number			
Money:			
• knows appropriate coins and notes for basic survival, e.g. phone, toilet, fares			
• adds up simple amounts, collects change			
Interacting with others:			
• behaves appropriately with strangers			
• uses basic social conversation, requests in shops, etc.			
• conforms to normal moral expectations, e.g.			
does not steal			
has appropriate sexual behaviour			

Community integration skills

	Can do without assistance	Can do with assistance	Cannot do
Movement in local and wider community:			
• knows local community			
• travels beyond neighbourhood			
• knows what to do if lost			
Travel:			
• uses buses, trains to get around			
Telephone:			
• uses private or public phone independently			
• knows how to use telephone directory ...			
• uses phone for social conversations			
• uses phone to obtain information			
• records emergency and frequently-used numbers			
Appearance:			
• adequate standard of personal grooming .			
• adequate standard of personal hygiene ...			
• dresses in sufficiently fashionable manner ...			
Money management:			
• knows value of notes and coins			
• adds up simple amounts of notes and coins			
• checks change correctly			
• saves for bills, household goods, clothes, etc.			
• knows how and when to pay bills			
• knows how to budget			
• knows how to use a bank			

	Can do without assistance	Can do with assistance	Cannot do

Shopping:
- knows appropriate shops for different goods ....
- locates items in shops ....
- attempts to compare prices ....
- interacts appropriately with shop assistants ....
- copes adequately with check-out systems ...

Community facilities:
- uses hairdresser when desired ....
- selects and purchases own clothes and other items ....
- knows how to use laundrette ....
- knows function of and can use post office, police, library, social security and other facilities ....

Personal competence:
- shows ability to be assertive when necessary ....
- understands what behaviour is illegal or socially offensive ....
- knows own clothing and shoe sizes ....
- aware of rights ....

Decision-making:
- plans outings and activities ....
- decides on meals, hobbies, routines ....
- shows awareness of and necessity for rules ....
- participates in decision-making in residence ....
- works out own solutions to problems .....
- votes ....

	Can do without assistance	Can do with assistance	Cannot do
Health:			
• makes appointments with GP, dentists, etc.			
• attends general practitioner and dentist when necessary			
• explains symptoms accurately			
• gets prescriptions dispensed			
Interacting with others:			
• demonstrates adequate social manners ...			
• introduces self to others appropriately			
• converses competently and appropriately in social situations			
• makes and retains friends of own choosing			
• aware of impact on others			
• aware of those who may exploit financially or sexually			
• shows consideration for neighbours and other tenants			
Personal relationships:			
• forms and maintains friendships			
• respects other people			
• aware of social standards for sexual behaviour			
• aware of birth control methods, ways of obtaining them and using them			
• knows causes and prevention of sexually transmitted diseases			
• understands implications of marital and other intimate relationships			
Literacy:			
• writes own name, address, phone number			
• fills in simple forms			

	Can do without assistance	Can do with assistance	Cannot do

Literacy: (contd.)
- makes simple lists ....
- prints simple messages ....

Domestic:
- pays rent regularly ....
- arranges for repairs to house and equipment ....
- shows some understanding of rental agreements ....

Leisure:
- able to use cinemas and theatres ....
- participates appropriately in community activities ....
- able to pursue leisure activities at home ....
- able to visit family and friends ....

Hospitality:
- prepares appropriately ....
- treats visitors appropriately ....
- provides appropriate food ....

Eating out:
- selects appropriate restaurant ....
- selects from menu ....
- understands role of waiter/waitress ....
- uses cutlery, glasses, etc., appropriately .....
- pays bill appropriately ....
- copes with alcohol appropriately ....

Need for programming
What are programs?
Basic steps in programming

7

Developing client skills: programming

Since the major goal of residential care is to meet the needs of individual clients, it is essential that helpers develop skills in providing appropriate forms of assistance. This chapter describes the way in which specific and individualised forms of help can be planned and implemented, that is, through programming. The chapter that follows explores some of the teaching strategies that can be used with programming and, in particular, programs relating to independent functioning and community integration.

NEED FOR PROGRAMMING

Most people acquire personal, interpersonal and social skills as a result of ongoing interactions in the everyday contexts in which they live and function. The basic learning process at work is an outcome of having learned how to learn, that is, having developed an ability to perceive situations, experiences and the actions of others in terms of a need to modify personal behaviour. When compared with the totality of a person's learning, the number of occasions beyond childhood when others consider it is necessary to point out learning needs, and to deliberately devise approaches to enable learning to take place, are relatively few.

The majority of disabled people are no different from others in the way in which they learn. Where helpers have the responsibility

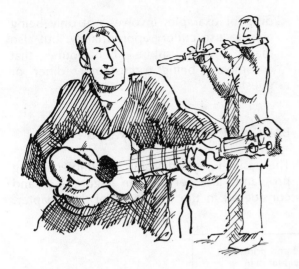

programming provides a framework for enabling them to learn how to become effective helpers.

WHAT ARE PROGRAMS?

In this book the term program is used in a specific way, that is:

> *a systematically organised, implemented and evaluated process aimed at developing specific client skills.*

Programs of this kind can be used to develop a wide range of skills including those relating to:

- personal care
- mobility
- self-awareness and personal identity
- group living
- functioning in mainstream society
- leisure, recreation and creativity.

Whatever the nature of programs that helpers wish to develop, it is important that programs are:

- chosen by clients
- consistent with what clients identify as their more important needs
- experienced by clients as helpful, enjoyable and as enhancing their feelings of self-worth

for the general patterning of their daily lives, the major orientation will be to ensure that all that happened promotes the acquisition of essential skills. The significance of the general quality of life in enabling clients to learn and develop normally cannot be overstressed, and it is a topic to which the third part of this book is devoted.

While the majority of clients have the potential to learn as a result of everyday events and transactions, it is nevertheless important that helpers acquire skills in implementing more formalised teaching approaches. Among the reasons why this should be so are that:

- there remains a group of clients, and particularly those with quite marked intellectual disabilities, who are unable to learn in the more usual ways. They are not capable of perceiving the cues in their environments or interactions with others that induce learning. Thus, for them, more formalised and consciously developed processes of learning are essential
- past approaches to disabled people, in assuming an incapacity to learn and develop, led to levels of neglect that left many entirely deficient in basic skills
- few helpers at present possess the expertise to ensure that clients develop necessary skills in the course of daily life, and so

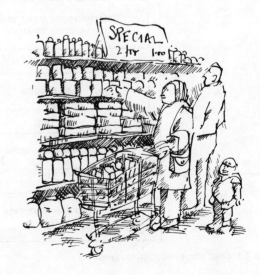

- related to needs detailed in individual plans
- based on a realistic appraisal of existing abilities and capacity to learn
- consistent with other forms of help being offered to clients
- carried out in contexts where there is consistency between what programs seek to achieve for clients and the general pattern of daily life
- able to achieve the development of appropriate role behaviour, of which specific skills are often aspects. Learning to dine

out, for example, involves not only being able to use cutlery appropriately, but also many more subtle behaviours that accompany being a customer, diner or guest.

BASIC STEPS IN PROGRAMMING

The basic steps in devising and implementing programs are set out in Figure 7.1 and considered in the remainder of this chapter.

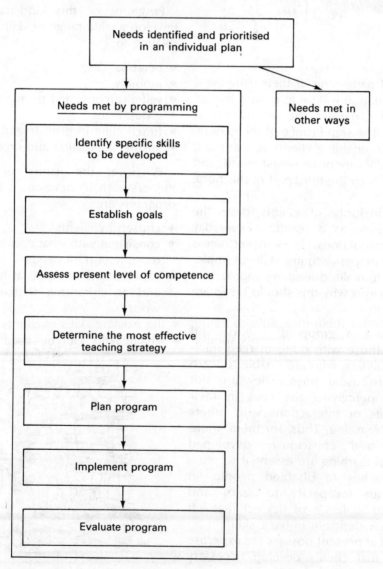

Fig. 7.1 Basic steps in programming.

While the impression may be given that all programs should be highly structured, that is not, in fact, the case. The degree of detail and exactness of each program will vary considerably according to such factors as the learning capacity of clients and skills to be learned.

Although this approach to developing client skills may at first seem complex and unnecessarily time-consuming, once helpers have achieved some basic competence in programming and clients have developed elementary participative skills, most of the stages become quite simple to work through and accomplish.

In summary, the stages in programming are:

Identifying skill to be developed
Establishing goals
Assessing present level of competence
Determining the most effective teaching strategies
Planning the program
Implementing the program
Evaluating the program.

Identifying skill to be developed

Decisions about skills to be developed will normally be related to the wishes of clients and needs identified in individual plans. Only in exceptional circumstances should programs be used to change the behaviour of clients without their knowledge and agreement. While it may appear that the disabilities of some clients render them incapable of being involved in decision-making, attempts should nevertheless be made to discuss help to be offered and to obtain client agreement.

Where clients have attended their own planning meetings they will already have agreed to the proposed programs. If, for any reason, they were excluded at the planning stage, decisions about programs should be discussed with them so that they:

- are able to understand the way others perceive their needs
- can state what they see as the more important skills to develop
- can comment on or disagree with the proposals of helpers
- can discuss the teaching strategies best suited to their needs.

Once there is agreement on the kinds of skills to be developed, it is necessary to prioritise them. Theoretically they should be developed in a logical sequence, that is, beginning with the client's existing skills and building on them to develop others. In reality, however, decisions about where to begin will be related to a number of other considerations such as:

- what clients see as their more important needs
- the kind of help necessary to make client rights a reality
- which programs are consistent with the daily life of clients
- which programs have the greatest chance of succeeding, thereby creating a climate of success and a base for future learning
- the existing skills of clients
- which skills can be used once they are developed
- which skills are basic to the development

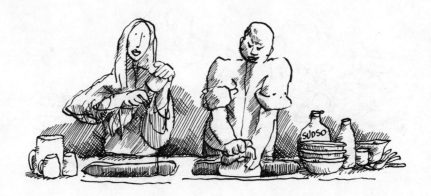

of other skills, for example, making a cup of tea as part of an overall goal of enabling clients to prepare breakfast, or being able to dress as part of a program of self-care
- the ability of helpers to use specific teaching approaches. This factor is particularly relevant for those residences where programming is at an elementary stage. In such residences it would probably be best to begin in a modest way and develop, as a result of minor successes, a sure and proven base from which to embark on more complex methods of helping.

Establishing goals

Having decided on the skill to be developed, it will be necessary to establish a formal goal for the program. This will be a general statement about what is to be accomplished. Goals are necessary because they:

- indicate, both for clients and helpers, what they are seeking to achieve
- provide a base for deciding the best teaching strategies
- serve as a basis for program evaluation.

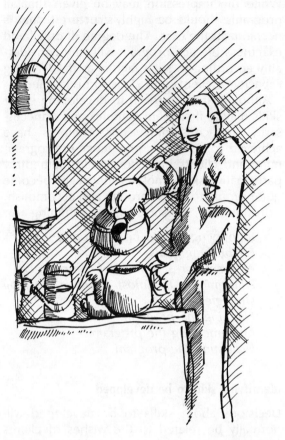

Assessing present level of competence

Before a program can be planned it is necessary to clarify to what extent the client is able to perform the skills in question. Available information may merely indicate that a client cannot perform the total skill and give no indication as to what he/she can actually do. The only way this kind of information can be obtained is by observing the client attempting the task. This is likely to involve making a record of the behaviour, and the most usual way of so doing is to break a task into its various stages and assess a client's competence at each stage. If, for example, a client is attempting to gain skills in the prep-

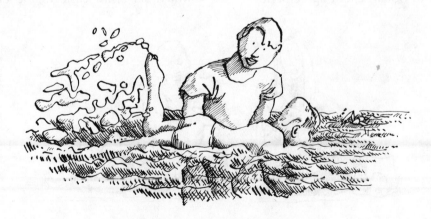

aration of meals and is to learn how to make a pot of tea, the extent of his/her present skill can be assessed by making a chart such as that in Table 7.1.

Table 7.1 Assessing skills: I

Stages in task	Can do without assistance	Can do with assistance	Cannot do
1. Gets out teapot and spoon			
2. Puts correct amount of tea/tea bags in pot			
3. Fills jug or kettle			
4. Boils water			
5. Pours water into pot			

As a second example, if a client wishes to learn how to wash his/her hair, that task can be broken down and assessed as in Table 7.2.

Table 7.2 Assessing skills: II

Stages in task	Can do without assistance	Can do with assistance	Cannot do
1. Wets hair			
2. Puts shampoo on hand			
3. Rubs shampoo into hair			
4. Rinses hair			
5. Dries hair			

For some clients and for some tasks it may be necessary to assess competence in a more detailed way. This can be achieved by undertaking a *task analysis* and using it to assess the clients' skills. A task analysis for teeth cleaning is given in Table 7.3.

It should be noted that developing and using such a task analysis is not a straight forward matter because:

- there will always be some disagreement over exactly how a task should be undertaken

- the many steps in even the most basic tasks indicate the kinds of difficulties severely disabled clients may experience in trying to accomplish them.

Table 7.3 Cleaning teeth: task analysis

Stages in task	Can do without assistance	Can do with assistance	Cannot do
1. Stand/sit in front of wash basin			
2. Turn cold tap on			
3. Pick up toothpaste			
4. Remove lid			
5. Put lid on top of wash basin			
6. Pick up tooth-brush			
7. Wet tooth-brush			
8. Squeeze toothpaste on to the brush			
9. Put toothpaste down			
10. Lift brush to mouth			
11. Brush top teeth outside front, up and down			
12. Brush top teeth outside left, up and down			
13. Brush top teeth outside right, up and down			
14. Brush top teeth inside front, up and down			
15. Brush top teeth inside left, up and down			
16. Brush top teeth inside right, up and down			
17. Brush bottom teeth outside front, up and down			
18. Brush bottom teeth outside left, up and down			
19. Brush bottom teeth outside right, up and down			

Table 7.3 (contd.)

Stages in task	Can do without assistance	Can do with assistance	Cannot do
20. Brush bottom teeth inside front, up and down			
21. Brush bottom teeth inside left, up and down			
22. Brush bottom teeth inside right, up and down			
23. Spit out toothpaste			
24. Rinse brush			
25. Put away brush			
26. Pick up cup			
27. Half fill with water			
28. Rinse mouth			
29. Spit out			
30. Put cup down			
31. Wipe mouth with towel			
32. Rinse cup			
33. Put cup away			
34. Replace lid of toothpaste			
35. Put toothpaste away			

In general, information gained by any method of assessment should provide:

- a fairly clear picture of the client's present ability
- information for establishing realistic program goals
- information about the number and kinds of stages that may be required in a program
- information about the overall way in which a program needs to be structured.

Determining the most effective teaching strategies

There are a number of ways of teaching skills to clients and some are discussed in the following chapter. In deciding which are the most appropriate for a particular program, the following factors should be considered:

- the wishes of clients. This will involve discussing with them how they can be helped and the advantages and disadvantages of different strategies
- learning abilities of clients
- teaching strategies staff are capable of implementing
- context in which learning is to take place
- resources available
- the advantages of group as against individual learning
- time and cost factors.

Planning the program

The next stage will be to plan the actual program. This will involve considering such issues as:

> Program objectives
> Equipment for the program
> Location of program
> Frequency of program
> Staff to run program
> Skill development
> Prompting the client
> Motivating the client.

Program objectives

The need for program goals has already been discussed. Some programs will require objectives as well as goals. Basically, objectives which are developed from goals, are much more precise statements about what is to be achieved and are necessary for determining the actual shape of programs, particularly those which need to be highly specific. Program objectives should, therefore:

- be expressed in precise language
- state exactly, in action terms, the skill to be developed, for example: 'The client will clean, brush, write . . .'
- be stated in ways that enable a client's response to be evaluated

- indicate what is to be used to determine success, for example:
  - the client will use the skill spontaneously on appropriate occasions
  - the client will be able to perform the skill when reminded
  - the client will accomplish the skill 80% of the time
  - for every ten attempts the client will succeed seven times
  - the skill will be sustained for three minutes.

A helpful way of stating objectives, where they lend themselves to it, will be to set them out as in Table 7.4.

Table 7.4 Program objectives

What the client will do
When
Where
In what way
Measure of success

Equipment for program

Some programs will require considerable equipment and materials and so they should be thought about and gathered together before a program is embarked upon. Whatever materials are needed should:

- be age appropriate
- be familiar to the client so as to avoid creating additional learning difficulties but, where appropriate, be sufficiently novel to stimulate interest
- enable skills learned to be transferred to other situations.

Location of program

Each program should be carried out in the most advantageous setting and, wherever possible and appropriate, be incorporated into the client's daily life. This is of particular importance for the development of normalised lifestyles.

Frequency of program

How often activities are carried out and the duration of sessions will be determined in relation to the skills to be learned, the learning capabilities of clients and the pattern of daily life.

Staff to run program

Among the factors to consider will be:

- numbers of staff needed to run a program
- helpers clients wish to assist them
- skills and abilities required of staff to operate programs effectively
- preparation and training of staff
- external help staff may need
- staff to evaluate programs.

Skill development

Many tasks include a mixture of simple and complex skills, and learning can often be enhanced by planning the way in which the various stages are to be presented. A task can be taught in different ways, for example:

- *Total task*: Each time clients work on a program they are encouraged to attempt the whole task and are helped with the particular stages with which they have difficulty.
- *Forward chaining*: Clients begin a program by working only on the first stage, with the rest of the task, where appropriate, being completed by clients and helpers together. When clients have learned the first stage they move on to the next one.
- *Reverse chaining*: Helpers and clients together complete the whole of the task with the exception of the last stage which is completed only by clients. Once that stage has been mastered clients work back through other stages.
- *Easy to difficult*: Most tasks will be made up of stages which differ in degrees of difficulty. It is sometimes helpful to teach the easier ones first and then work through others in terms of increasing difficulty,

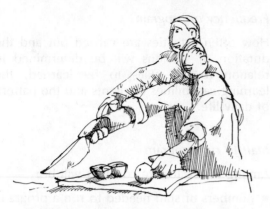

finally joining them together in their logical sequence.

Prompting the client

An important aspect of any form of instruction is to provide learners, as they attempt tasks, with cues about what it is they should be doing, and this is known as prompting. There are three forms of prompting, the use of which will be related to a client's learning abilities, the skill in question and the stage of the program. The three forms of prompting are:

- *Physical prompting*: The helper physically guides the actions of clients until they become aware of what they should be doing.

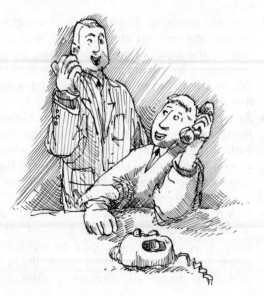

- *Verbal prompting*: The helper prompts the client by giving short, verbal, matter-of-fact statements immediately before the client attempts the desired behaviour; for example, 'Move it up and down', 'Put it under the tap', 'Pour the water in the pot', 'Try it now'.
- *Non-verbal prompting*: In addition, or as an alternative to verbal prompting, the helper can use gestures such as beckoning or pointing.

Motivating the client

However well-intentioned a person may be, acquiring new skills as a result of programming is never easy. It is a process that essentially involves considerable self-discipline to overcome the difficulties, embarrassment and failures encountered in the course of learning.

A significant way of reducing these difficulties is to motivate learners by rewarding them with something they desire when their efforts are successful. In the context of programming, rewards can be in the form of events, objects, food or activities, or they can be inherent in the task. They can be provided by helpers working on the program with the client or they can originate elsewhere. Finally, they can be given to clients before, during or after learning.

Among the specific forms of motivation helpers can use when assisting clients acquire new skills are:

- *Encouragement and demonstration of approval*: That is, acknowledging success through appropriate praise, warm gestures and touch.
- *Tangible rewards*: These will be items desired by clients and those which are not usual or necessary aspects of daily life. Whatever tangible rewards are used should be age appropriate and be accompanied by approval. Among tangible rewards that can be used are drinks, sweets and activities, and also tokens which can be exchanged for other desired items.

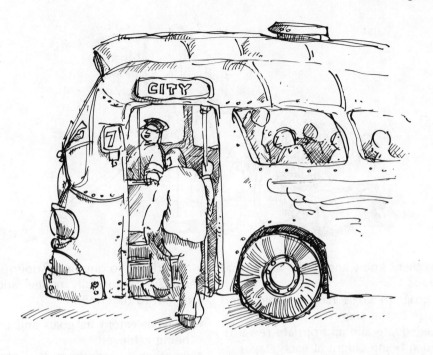

Probably the best forms of motivation are those which are natural, that is, where learners get pleasure from attempting and succeeding at the task or where they make an effort as a result of the encouragement of others. There can be a number of problems associated with tangible rewards in that they can create dependence and so make it difficult for the learner to learn without them. It is the case, however, that many disabled people, and particularly those with marked intellectual disabilities, have difficulty in learning in the usual ways and so do not respond to the more natural forms of motivation. For this group tangible rewards may be essential.

The most effective forms of motivation can be ascertained by:

- asking clients how they wish to be rewarded
- observing and trying to identify preferences
- experimenting with different rewards.

When using rewards it is important to ensure that they:

- have positive consequences for clients
- are available at the agreed time
- are used consistently by all helpers involved in a program.

Implementing a program

However well a program has been planned, once in operation it may not run at all smoothly. There may be clear indications from clients that they are experiencing difficulties or are not enjoying what they are doing. They may, for example:

- continually avoid working on the program
- be easily distracted
- refuse to co-operate
- get worse rather than better at completing the various stages
- increasingly resort to inappropriate behaviour when the program is in operation
- fail to be motivated by the rewards offered.

Whatever the client's response, the most constructive initial reaction is to view the program itself as faulty. The following questions may help to identify what is wrong and thus lead to appropriate changes:

- Is the program too difficult or too easy in its present form?

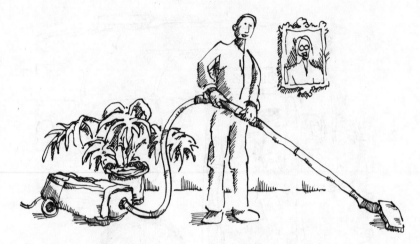

- Does the client know and understand what is expected?
- Do the program goals have meaning and make sense to the client?
- Is there adequate and appropriate reward?
- Is too much being taught at each stage?
- Are expectations for the rate of learning realistic?
- Is the program moving too quickly or not quickly enough?
- Does it bore the client?
- Can the client see that it is likely to have a worthwhile result?
- Is the program being run consistently?
- Are program sessions too long or too short?
- Are difficulties being caused in the environment in which the program is being carried out?
- Are the actions of staff creating problems?

Evaluating the program

As clients work on programs their progress should be monitored so that any necessary changes can be made to improve the rate of learning. This evaluation can be achieved:

- by using a checklist on which client responses can be recorded
- through direct observation
- through discussion with clients.

It is always of value to involve clients in monitoring programs and so it will be necessary to record progress in a way that makes sense to them.

In addition to ongoing monitoring, it will be necessary to formally review and evaluate a program to determine:

- to what extent its goals and objectives are being achieved
- whether to continue the program in its present form
- whether to abandon the program entirely.

These issues should be considered at some point because it is unfair for clients to be subjected to programs on an indefinite basis, and certainly to ones which may never be successfully completed.

A program can be considered a success if:

- a client is able to perform the skill
- a client has reached his/her ability level
- a client can perform the skill in settings different from that in which the program was carried out
- skills learned can be generalised, for example, filling a glass for the purpose of rinsing the mouth after teeth cleaning, to filling a cup to obtain a drink
- a client is able to undertake the skill where there is some variation in instruction.

Finally, once a program has been successfully completed it may be appropriate to:

- detail how, when and where the client can use the skill
- identify the next skill to work on
- suggest a time for reviewing client use of new skills.

Interactive learning
Instruction
Demonstration
Role play
Behaviour modification

8

Developing client skills: teaching strategies

The preceding chapter describes in a general way the planning and implementation of programs. This chapter details some of the teaching strategies helpers can use when running programs, and particularly those which aim at developing the kinds of skills detailed in the checklist in Chapter 6.

The extent to which clients are able to learn as a result of programming is dependent upon the use of appropriate teaching strategies. The reasons why this should be so are, firstly, many clients are likely to find this kind of learning quite difficult. They may, for example:

- have had no previous experience of programming
- not have had experience of relating to helpers as teachers
- lack motivation and commitment to learning
- have little confidence that much can be accomplished.

Secondly, a significant proportion of the skills clients will be attempting to develop are quite complex ones. An examination of the checklist in Chapter 6 indicates that many are not simply about the performance of precise skills, such as washing dishes or making telephone calls, but essentially concern role behaviour, that is, patterns of behaviour appropriate to social contexts such as a diner in a restaurant, patient in a dentist's surgery and customer in shops. While such roles involve a number of quite specific behaviours, they are at the same time complex, dynamic and variable, thus making it impossible to

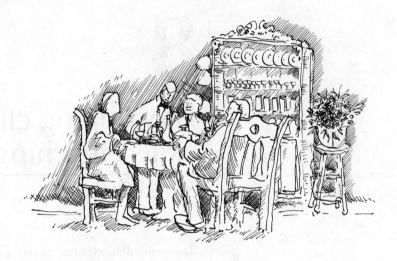

state for learning purposes the precise behaviour involved. The role, for example, of passenger on a bus, while necessitating the ability to get on and off at the required stops, paying the fare and finding a seat, also involves more subtle behaviours that will be an outcome of travelling at a certain time of the day or week, on a particular route and in the company of particular drivers and passengers. Successful performance of roles requires of individuals the ability to monitor both their own actions and those of others, and to anticipate what is likely to occur so that they can adjust their behaviour accordingly. Skills of this kind can only be acquired in learning situations that present to the learner experiences that are similar to those of real life situations.

The teaching strategies discussed in this chapter range from those which lend themselves to the development of quite specific skills to those relating to social roles. They are:

> *Interactive learning*
> *Instruction*
> *Demonstration*
> *Role play*
> *Behaviour modification.*

It should be noted that these strategies are not alternatives; where complex skills are involved at least two are likely to be employed. Furthermore, while the major goal in using these strategies will be to develop client skills, an equally important additional goal will be the attainment of greater self-esteem, self-confidence and a stronger awareness of personal identity. Finally, whatever strategies are used should be in the context of relationships which clients value and experience as supportive.

When developing programs and selecting teaching strategies a number of factors should be considered such as:

- the strategies clients consider will best enable them to learn
- the learning abilities of clients
- what appear to be the more appropriate strategies for specific skills
- the degree of complexity of the skills in question
- the ability of helpers to use particular teaching strategies
- the contexts in which a program is to be undertaken.

INTERACTIVE LEARNING

Interactive learning is the way in which most people in the normal course of life develop personal and social skills. In residential contexts, as helpers become more aware of client need and develop abilities in creating positive helping environments, this is likely to become the main mode of learning.

Interactive learning uses everyday situations and relationships to enable clients to learn. Essentially, learning takes place as a result of structuring, or shaping, usual daily contacts and events so that clients are able to acquire skills in quite normal ways. Where, for example, a client is to learn the skill of bed making, he/she can do so by making his/her bed with a helper at the appropriate time each day. As they attempt the task the helper explains and demonstrates what the client should be doing. The helper may say, 'Go round the other side of the bed. Now, get hold of the top covers like this, don't touch the bottom sheet for a moment, and pull the covers back with me.' And a second example, if a client is to learn how to care for his/her clothes the helper may suggest the two of them tidy the client's wardrobe, drawers or cupboard together. As they do so, the helper will point out which items are best kept together, how clothes can be hung or folded and which items appear to require washing or cleaning.

Despite the informal nature of this approach it nevertheless requires thought and planning along the lines indicated in the previous chapter, not only to decide which skills can be taught in this way but how each part of a skill can be presented.

INSTRUCTION

Most clients will be able to develop many skills as a result of formal instruction. As the word 'formal' implies, this is a method of instruction, very much like that which takes place in the school, where either individuals or groups receive directions and explanations about what they are to learn. In the context of work with disabled people it is a method of teaching that will be successful where:

- clients are able to comprehend what is being taught
- clients have the ability to cope with formal learning situations and are willing participants

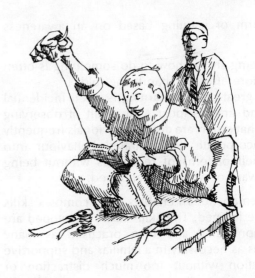

- client learning can be maximised by this method.

Even though this form of teaching is quite formal in terms of presentation of material, it should nevertheless take place in a warm and relaxed atmosphere where the boundaries between clients and helpers are not marked and where positive interaction and continuous discussion can occur.

DEMONSTRATION

Demonstration involves a client observing someone performing the behaviour to be learned and then attempting to imitate it. It is

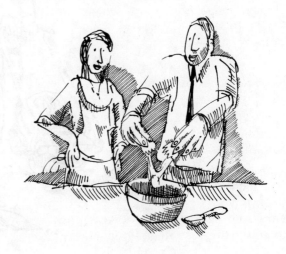

a form of learning based on an awareness that:

- being shown how to do something is often more effective than being told
- a great deal of learning is often incidental and unconscious. As a result of observing what others are doing, individuals frequently incorporate demonstrated behaviour into their patterns of responses without being aware of what has happened.

Demonstration enables quite complex skills to be learned. The skills to be developed are demonstrated and then practised as many times as necessary in a familiar and supportive situation without too much distraction or embarrassment.

This method of learning is appropriate for clients who:

- can understand what is involved in the demonstration process
- are able to observe with considerable accuracy the demonstrated behaviour
- can imitate demonstrated behaviour.

Demonstration process

In a context which has been suitably prepared and which is as natural and normal as possible, the behaviour to be learned is demonstrated in total, and in a way that can be understood by the client. It is then repeated one or more times with an explanation and discussion of each step, emphasising the more difficult aspects. This will enable the client to clarify any difficulties and confusions and to know what he/she should be observing.

Following a client's attempts to imitate the behaviour the helper and client can discuss what took place to:

- highlight what went on, who did what, what was said, and the consequences of specific actions
- identify feelings and attitudes that accompany the demonstrated behaviour
- identify appropriate social contexts in which the behaviour in question can be used.

ROLE PLAY

As the term itself implies, role play is a form of learning that focuses on the development of skills integral to role performance, and it is highly effective in enabling disabled people to

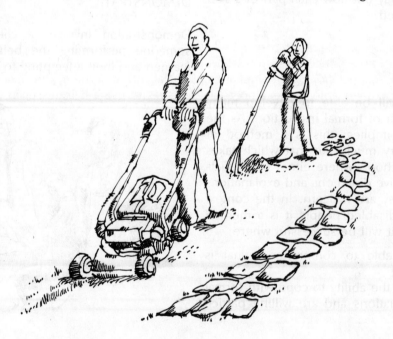

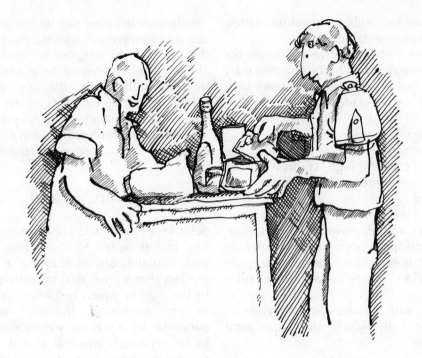

acquire skills for more normalised functioning.

A large number of those disabled people who have lived for many years in residential facilities are not able to behave appropriately in social roles. The isolated and sheltered nature of their lifestyles has provided them with few opportunities for experiencing social roles other than that of patient, inmate or resident. Furthermore, since these roles have been based on expectations of compliance, clients have not been able to develop basic interaction skills essential for social functioning. When faced with new situations in mainstream society, not only do they experience difficulty in coping with and relating to others, they often have little awareness of their own inadequacies. Whilst it would appear reasonable to expect them to learn through a process of trial and error, the difficulty they face is that as soon as others in mainstream society experience their behaviour as inappropriate or abnormal they make allowances and treat disabled people as special, so tending to reinforce inappropriate behaviour. Additionally, of course, for disabled people lacking social skills, mainstream society can be a quite hostile and unsympathetic context for learning. Thus, it is often essential that at least some initial learning takes place in specially prepared environments.

Role play is essentially learning by doing; it is about the creation of artificial situations and contexts in which clients can practise and learn the kinds of behaviour associated with social roles. Where, for example, a client wishes to use a hairdresser in the community and has never done so before, a simulated situation can be created in a residence that will enable him/her to become familiar with some of the exchanges that will take place. This may include discussing styles with the hairdresser and co-operating with requests, observing and commenting on the style when the job has been completed and paying for the service. As a result of such an experience the client will be sufficiently familiar with what is involved to have considerable chance of behaving appropriately in a real situation.

In summary, successful role play enables clients to:

- acquire complex skills in a holistic rather than a compartmentalised way
- learn in safe and supportive environments which are minimally embarrassing and least inhibiting, that is, where no problems arise when mistakes are made and where opportunities exist for trial and error learning without negative consequences
- learn at an appropriate pace because the time scale can, through control of the learning environment, be extended or compressed
- appreciate the subtleties, feelings and expectations accompanying role behaviour
- learn to anticipate both their own behaviour and that of others, and to appreciate the extent to which behaviour in roles varies
- experiment with variations in behaviour to find those with which they are most comfortable.

Role play process

As was the case with learning through demonstration, a setting should be prepared beforehand to make it as authentic as possible. Once this had been done, a number of stages need to be worked through:

> *Stage one*: Ensure that the client is aware of what is to happen and what he/she has to do, that is, how to behave, what to look for, cues for behaviour and what to anticipate.
> *Stage two*: Enact the role play, either in part or in total, and provide helpful comments, suggestions and prompts along the way.
> *Stage three*: On completion of a particular step or the whole of a role play, discuss with the client what took place including the nature of interactions, who said what to whom, who did what, language and tone of voice used, cues given to those involved, feelings accompanying particular interactions.
> *Stage four*: Repeat the role play until client feels relatively confident.

Role play learning can be enhanced by the use of role reversal, that is, the client taking the role, not of self, but of others involved. This enables him/her to be aware of the way in whch others are thinking, feeling and acting. Role play can also involve the use of video, film, illustrations of people in specific situations, and discussions with clients of past experiences or imaginary situations.

BEHAVIOUR MODIFICATION

Behaviour modification is a method of instruction that is suited to those who experience particular difficulty in learning. It is built on the fact that a great deal of learning is related to the way in which behaviour is responded to and reinforced. In other words, if a particular act is positively reinforced it is likely to be repeated, whereas if it is ignored or negatively reinforced it is unlikely to be repeated. Thus, if, for example, a parent wishes to teach a child to use a knife appropriately at mealtimes, approving of, or rewarding, the correct behaviour is likely to result in the child using the knife appropriately on subsequent occasions. Also, if the child is ignored for inappropriate use, he/she will be more likely in the future to use it in the desired way.

Some prior considerations

Many helpers assisting disabled people object to behaviour modification. Among the arguments they use are:

- the assumptions it makes about how people learn are too simplistic, that is, that present behaviour is not always the result of past reinforcement
- the manipulation of people by the use of reward and punishment is degrading and cannot be justified
- the attitudes towards disabled people implicit in the behaviour modification approach are out of step with the value accorded them by contemporary society

- little differentiation is made between human and animal learning and thus, by implication, this approach denies the uniqueness of humans, the ability to attribute meaning to behaviour and the acceptance of personal responsibility for behaviour.

Whatever the validity of these objections, it remains a fact that a great deal of learning takes place as a result of reinforcement. The behaviour of children growing up in the family, for example, is shaped by the way their parents reinforce what they do, and the behaviour of adults in the work situation is considerably affected by the actions of colleagues or more senior workers. Perhaps the only difference between this form of reinforcement learning and that used in behaviour modification programs is that the latter involves formal, contrived approaches whereas the former relies on more spontaneous everyday interactions. Since this is the case, disputes over behaviour modification as a process of instruction should not be about its use, but about the point at which a particular program goes beyond what is considered as desirable and acceptable.

Behaviour modification programs

Behaviour modification programs are suited to clients who are not able to learn in the more natural and incidental ways, and so they emphasise systematic use of reinforcement. The general shape of a program will be consistent with the overall framework discussed in Chapter 7. Each stage will be carefully and precisely planned and put into action. Thus:

- assessment of a client's present level of competence should be thorough
- clear objectives for a program should be set
- the task should be broken down into as many stages as appear necessary
- each stage should be carefully planned
- the use of reinforcement to increase learning should be tightly controlled.

Information relating to the first four of these points has been explored in Chapter 7 and the remainder of this section will consider the

fourth point, that is, the use of reinforcement to maximise learning.

Positive reinforcement

Experience with the use of reinforcement demonstrates that it is not always necessary to reinforce appropriate behaviour on every occasion. Individuals motivated by reinforcement usually respond in anticipation of rewards so long as they are received when expected. Thus reinforcement should be planned and used according to a clearly understood schedule. There are two basic forms reinforcement can take:

- *continuous reinforcement*: the client is rewarded every time he/she responds appropriately
- *intermittent reinforcement*: the client is rewarded on certain occasions. There are four forms of intermittent reinforcement:
  - fixed interval: the reward is given to the client after he/she has responded appropriately for a specific time period, for example, every three minutes
  - fixed ratio: the reward is given to the client after he/she responded appropriately a set number of times, for example, every fifth time
  - variable interval: the client is rewarded at planned but varying intervals, for example after two, then five, then ten minutes
  - variable ratio: the client is rewarded after a set but varying number of responses, for example, after the first, third, and sixth occasion.

When clients begin to work on quite difficult tasks they may not be able to perform them accurately whatever the rewards. To deny a reward until an acceptable standard is attained can destroy motivation and so clients' attempts that approximate to the desired behaviour should be reinforced. As they become more skilled, the level of accuracy expected of them can be increased. Additionally, once the client is working successfully on a program, the use of tangible reinforcers can be decreased and replaced by more natural forms of reinforcement.

Items used to reinforce behaviour should be those which:

- can be given immediately
- can be given regularly and repeatedly
- are desired by the client
- are appropriate to the client.

Where a client is not responding positively to a behaviour modification program, in addition to considering the questions listed in the previous chapter, it may be necessary to:

- vary the rate of reinforcement
- introduce different forms of reinforcement.

Negative reinforcement

A second form of reinforcement is negative reinforcement. This is a difficult concept to understand and often causes much confusion. Basically negative reinforcement involves the removal of certain events that are inhibiting the individual from responding in the desired way. As a result of their removal the desired or appropriate behaviour is strengthened.

Negative reinforcement is frequently confused with punishment. The two are quite different. The former, as has been suggested, involves the removal of something to achieve the desired behaviour, whereas the latter involves the addition of something unpleasant. From the point of view of behaviour modification programs, punishment is undesirable because it suppresses rather than eliminates unacceptable behaviour. A more general discussion of punishment is included in Chapter 16.

Good client records
Policy for client records
Range of documentation

9

Client records

Record keeping has often been viewed as an unpleasant and time-consuming task which, while being necessary to meet certain organisational requirements, has little to do with actually helping clients. This view is not without some justification in that client records in many residential settings are little more than repositories for vast amounts of paper, most of which is unrelated to client need or helping processes.

It has sometimes been the case that while records have been well kept, they have not served the interests of clients. In the past, for example, records have often:

- accumulated and reinforced critical and judgemental opinions about clients
- served to substantiate particular theoretical orientations
- complicated helping because of an expectation of comprehensive but quite unnecessary documentation
- been used to rationalise client behaviour in ways that make the activities of helpers appear positive
- translated observations into fact
- provided helpers with excuses for being in offices and away from clients
- been used by staff as symbols of power over clients
- over-formalised helping processes so making them mystifying to clients.

Maintaining good records in residential facilities is an essential dimension of the

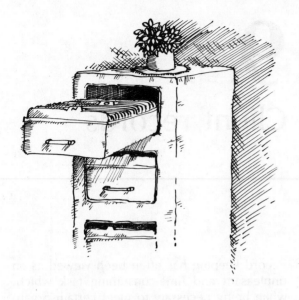

helping process. Recording and retaining a range of information about clients is important for many reasons such as:

- identifying need, setting goals, planning and reviewing helping processes
- devising and operating programs
- keeping a permanent record of significant events such as visits, accidents or illnesses
- informing others assisting clients of what is being attempted and what has been achieved
- enabling helpers to be accountable for their actions.

GOOD CLIENT RECORDS

If records are to be useful they will be:

- *Confidential*: People not involved in assisting clients or who have no need or right to see records should not have access to them.
- *Accessible*: Records should be readily available to all entitled to read and use them including the client.
- *Client centred*: Information recorded and retained in files will relate only to the needs of clients.
- *Positive*: A useful record will describe a client's total life situation in terms of strengths and not just weaknesses.
- *Jargon free*: A conscious attempt should be

made to exclude unnecessary technical terminology.
- *Succinct*: Records should contain only useful information and be as brief as possible.
- *Structured*: A record should be arranged in logical sequence and kept well-organised.
- *Identifiable*: Those making written contributions to records should identify themselves and date their entries.
- *Challengeable*: All people involved in helping clients, as well as clients themselves, their close relatives and advocates, should be able to question what has been recorded and, where appropriate, have unacceptable entries altered or deleted.
- *Kept up to date*: Records where the most recent information is many weeks old are of little use.
- *Accurate*: A statement purporting to be factual should be. This does not exclude either the expression of feeling or unsubstantiated comment, but where entries of this kind are made it should be clear that they are not factual.
- *Reflect the views of clients and their close relatives*: Thus they should be able to make their own entries.

POLICY FOR CLIENT RECORDS

Organisations assisting disabled people should develop policies and procedures governing the use of records. These will detail:

- the kinds of records to be kept
- information to be recorded, in what form and by whom
- confidentiality and accessibility
- storage of records, for example, in a central file, in the residences in which clients live, or a mix of both
- the way information can be used
- period of time various kinds of information should be retained.

RANGE OF DOCUMENTATION

A number of draft forms are set out in the

following pages to suggest the kind of documentation organisations assisting disabled people may wish to use. Each is best viewed as a starting point and as conveying ideas rather than an actual form to be used. The forms included have the following titles:

Personal information
Request for residential assistance
Residential services: intake information
Admission information
Individual plans
Client diary.

PERSONAL INFORMATION		Page 1.
NAME:		
DATE OF BIRTH:	SEX:	
MARITAL STATUS:		
IDENTIFYING CHARACTERISTICS:		
Height:	PHOTOGRAPH	
Weight:		
Colour of hair:		
Colour of eyes:		
Complexion:		
Ethnic origin:		
Distinguishing features:		
Brief description of client		
Details of disability and its consequences for client:		
Home Address:	Phone Number:	
Present Residence:	Phone Number:	
Next of Kin:	Phone Number:	
Advocate or other contact:	Phone Number:	

PERSONAL INFORMATION   Page 2.

PREVIOUS PLACEMENTS IN RESIDENTIAL ACCOMMODATION:

Residence	Reasons	Date of Entry	Date of Leaving

OTHER SERVICES RECEIVED:

Agency	Service	Date of Commencement	Date of Leaving

PERSONAL HISTORY:

Details of Family:

	Date of Birth	Present Residence	Additional Information
Father			
Mother			
Other Relevant Adults			
Siblings			

MEDICAL INFORMATION:

Doctors & Specialists Involved:

Details of Disabilities:

Recurrent Illnesses:

PERSONAL INFORMATION			Page 3.

PERSONAL HISTORY (Contd.)

DETAILS OF PREVIOUS ASSISTANCE TO CLIENT & FAMILY:

| Services | Dates | | Reason |
	From	To	

EDUCATION INFORMATION:

Name of School	Dates	Comments

EMPLOYMENT INFORMATION:

Employer	Dates	Comments

REQUEST FOR RESIDENTIAL ASSISTANCE
(* See note)

	Date of Application:

Surname of Client:	Given Names:

Date of Birth:	Sex:	Marital Status:

Home Address:	Post Code:
	Phone Number:

Present Address (if different):	Post Code:
	Phone Number:

Name of Person Making Application:	Designation:

Employing Body, Address:	Post Code:
	Phone Number:

PREVIOUS OR PRESENT SERVICES TO CLIENT AND FAMILY:

OTHER AGENCIES INVOLVED:

REASONS FOR REFERRAL:

SERVICES OR HELP REQUIRED:

SUMMARY OF DECISIONS MADE:

* <u>Note</u>: This form is to be completed by the person making the request for residential care prior to an intake meeting.

RESIDENTIAL SERVICES : INTAKE INFORMATION   Page 1.
(* See note i)

Surname of Client:	Given Names:

Date of Birth:	Sex:	Marital Status:

Home Address:	Post Code:
	Phone Number:
Present Address (if different):	Post Code:
	Phone Number

ALLOCATION TEAM:

	Organisation	Involvement with Client
Chairperson:		
Others Attending:		
Person Making Referral:		

REASONS FOR REFERRAL:

SUMMARY OF DISCUSSION:

IDENTIFIED NEEDS:

DECISION (See note ii)

RESIDENTIAL SERVICES : INTAKE INFORMATION   Page 2.

NEEDS TO BE MET BY RESIDENTIAL SERVICES:

ASSISTANCE TO BE PROVIDED:

Action	Persons Responsible

PREPARATION PROGRAM:

Steps	Action	Persons Responsible

Proposed Date of Admission

* Notes i: This form is to be completed by the chairperson or some other appropriate person and is a formal summary of the intake meeting.

    ii: Where the decision is against admitting a client to residential care, information should be given about other services that should be made available.

```
┌─────────────────────────────────────────────────────────────────┐
│                    ADMISSION INFORMATION                          │
├───────────────────────────────┬───────────────────────────────────┤
│ Surname of Client:            │ Given Names                       │
├───────────────────────────────┼───────────────────────────────────┤
│ Date of Admission:            │ Likely Duration of Stay:          │
├───────────────────────────────┴───────────────────────────────────┤
│ Unit or Residence Client Admitted to:                             │
│                                                                   │
├───────────────────────────────────────────────────────────────────┤
│ Health Needs:                                                     │
│                                                                   │
├───────────────────────────────────────────────────────────────────┤
│ Personal Care Requirements:                                       │
│                                                                   │
├───────────────────────────────────────────────────────────────────┤
│ Medication:                                                       │
│                                                                   │
├───────────────────────────────────────────────────────────────────┤
│ Other Needs:                                                      │
│                                                                   │
├───────────────────────────────────────────────────────────────────┤
│ Person to Contact in an Emergency:                                │
│                                                                   │
└───────────────────────────────────────────────────────────────────┘
```

INDIVIDUAL PLANS (See note i)		**PLAN NUMBER:** _____ (See note ii)

Name of Client:
Home Address:
Residence:

Date of Birth:	Date of Admission:

PLANNING TEAM:

Member	Designation
Chairperson:	
Key Worker:	

REVIEW OF PREVIOUS PLAN:

Need	Extent to which Need was Met
1.	
2.	
3.	
4.	
5.	

GENERAL OBSERVATIONS ABOUT NEEDS:

INDIVIDUAL PLANS (cont.)   Page 2.

LONGER TERM AND IMMEDIATE NEEDS:

NEEDS FOR ACTION: (See Note iii)

Need	Action	By Whom
1.		
2.		
3.		
4.		
5.		

ADDITIONAL INFORMATION REQUIRED RELATING TO IMMEDIATE NEEDS:

CLIENT'S CONSENT TO PLAN:

DATE OF NEXT REVIEW:

Notes: (i)   to be completed by key worker, plan co-ordinator or other
               relevant person.

        (ii)   the number of plan, i.e. if it is the first, second, etc.,
               should be inserted.

        (iii) should include needs such as accommodation, education,
               family support and assistance, work, leisure and personal
               help.

	CLIENT DIARY (See note)	
Date	Entry	Signature

Note: A log of this kind will be kept for all clients in a residence.

It will record important information, for example:

.   sickness

.   visits

.   unusual or significant events

.   problems

.   relevant comments

PART | THREE

Normalising
residential life

Over the past twenty years a great deal of criticism has been made of the residential facility as a context for assisting disabled people. In looking at the various explanations for poor residential services, it is surprising to note that little attention has been given to the quality of the residential environment and the nature of daily life. It is as if what happens to disabled people on a day-to-day basis is seen to be unrelated to the lives they live and the people they become.

The nature of the living environment is probably the single most important factor that determines client experiences, and the one that needs greatest attention. The shape it takes is a consequence of worker attitudes and practices, and the pattern of life workers create for clients. Without an appreciation of its importance, and the provision of a client-centred way of life, disabled people will continue to be seriously handicapped by the very services that are supposed to exist to assist them.

The following seven chapters offer a range of ideas for thinking about and improving residential life. An underlying belief is that most residential contexts have the potential to meet the needs of clients where they are structured and operated on a client-centred basis. Chapter 10 explores many of the more important dimensions that contribute to the quality of daily life, particularly factors relating to the living environment, patterns of relationships and the daily routine. Chapter 11 discusses small community residences, their significance in terms of future service provision and the ways in which they can be established and maintained. Chapter 12 looks at the part parents and relatives of disabled people can play in residential life. Chapter 13 discusses ways of integrating disabled people into mainstream society, and the contribution volunteers are able to make. Chapter 14 explores the needs of disabled children, adolescents and aged people, and chapter 15 considers issues relating to education, work and leisure. Finally, Chapter 16 looks at ways in which problem behaviour can be understood and responded to in the residential environment.

A setting in which to live
A setting in which to grow
A setting for greater independence
A setting for meaningful relationships
A setting for normal daily life

10

Creating a beneficial residential environment

Of the many factors influencing the quality of life in residential accommodation, perhaps the most significant are a consequence of the way the living environment is structured. The nature of the environment influences, if not determines:

- the day-to-day experiences of clients
- the extent to which their basic needs are met
- the quality of their relationships with others
- the degree of independence they are able to enjoy
- the extent to which their lives are normalised.

Whatever helpers seek to achieve for clients through specialised forms of assistance makes little sense and cannot be justified if clients live in detrimental environments. Thus a prerequisite for all forms of assistance is a living context which, in being client centred, meets basic needs. It is important to acknowledge that such an environment should not be viewed simply as one of a number of ways of assisting disabled people; it is a right and should exist irrespective of what may be sought for them in specific areas of their lives.

This chapter discusses a number of dimensions that are common to most forms of residential life and which affect the nature of client experiences. While many of the ideas included have obvious relevance for larger, congregate facilities, they are also pertinent to smaller ones. There is clear evidence to indicate that size in itself does not determine the quality of residential life; not only can a small residence be just as institutional as a large one, a larger facility can be as personalised as a smaller one.

The ideas in this chapter are organised under five broad headings each of which focuses on certain dimensions of need. They explore residential care as a setting:

> *In which to live*
> *In which to grow*
> *For greater independence*
> *For meaningful relationships*
> *For normal daily life.*

A SETTING IN WHICH TO LIVE

Residential care as home

Whatever else residential care seeks to offer to disabled people, the residence in which they live should be seen primarily as their home. That is not to assert that, if they have a home elsewhere, the residence should be thought of as their only home, nor as the central and most important base for living their lives, but that it should:

- offer a pattern of life that can be identified as home-like
- provide the pleasant experiences and security most people enjoy when living at home

- be experienced by clients as home on both a feeling and an emotional level.

What are the dimensions associated with home that should be reflected in a residence? In general, a home-like context offers clients opportunities for:

- safety, protection and security
- small group living
- determining the pattern of daily life
- developing feelings of belonging and group identity.

While residential facilities for adults will seek to be home-like, there should be no attempt to model them on family life in mainstream society or operate them in similar ways. There are significant differences between family and group living and the two should not be confused. The pattern of life in most families is built upon unequal relationships between adults and children, and the use by parents of their power to shape living arrangements and interactions. In residential situations where groups of adult people live, staff should not act as if they were parents; to do so is to impose an inappropriate lifestyle on clients. Furthermore, the obligations and interactions that characterise sibling relationships in the family involve quite special freedoms but at the same time clear limitations. Since clients are not siblings, it is wrong for

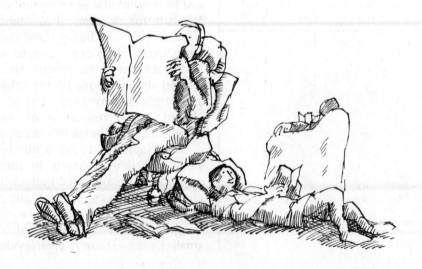

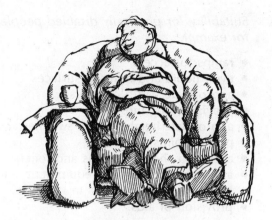

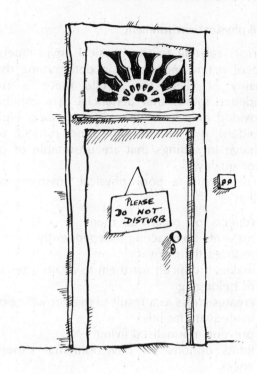

helpers to expect them to function as if they were.

If a home-like living environment is to be attained, both staff and clients should be selected:

- on the basis of their likely compatibility with the existing group
- because of their desire to become a member of the group
- because of the group's desire to have them as a member. This means that the group should control the selection of new members, both clients and staff
- with the understanding that no member will be moved from the group merely for oganisational convenience.

Privacy

Privacy is recognised as a basic need, and it is an aspect of life that is often absent in many residences. In practice privacy means:

- being able to go somewhere to get away from or be with others
- exercising choice about being on one's own or with others
- having opportunities to withdraw from interaction with others
- being able to deal with bodily needs and functions and to dress and undress in a dignified way without an audience
- not having to reveal all personal details, thoughts and feelings.

It can be attained by:

- recognising the need for privacy, and individual differences in the extent to which it is desired
- providing single bedrooms which clients can lock
- establishing an understanding that staff and clients knock before entering rooms
- individualising shower, bath and toilet times and minimising intrusion and assistance
- helpers seeking permission before carrying out personal caring tasks for clients
- permitting greater freedom within a residential facility and beyond it
- enabling clients to spend more time on their own and with people of their own choosing
- providing telephones in suitable locations so that clients can make and receive calls in private
- ensuring that confidentiality governs the sending and receiving of mail.

The physical environment

Factors relating to the physical environment are of major importance in determining the quality of client life. While there is no evidence to say that beneficial care can be provided only in facilities that are of a high standard, it is, at the same time, difficult to achieve in settings that are unsuitable or of poor quality.

For clients, a poor physical environment often:

- reflects low regard for them
- prevents them acting independently
- reduces their privacy
- makes it difficult for them to attain a sense of belonging
- creates stress as a result of overcrowding or inadequate facilities
- prevents normalised living
- limits options for developmental experiences.

for staff it can:

- make their task difficult and provide little opportunity for satisfying work experiences
- have a negative effect on morale
- make them defensive about, and sometimes ashamed of, where they work
- contribute to the stress they experience.

A good residential care environment will reflect a number of desirable features such as:

Suitability for physically disabled people, for example:

- ramps for access
- even floors and non-slip surfaces
- appropriate width of doors
- provision of hand rails
- appropriate height of light switches and power points
- access to showers, baths and toilets
- appropriate siting of equipment and height of work benches in kitchens
- provision of aids.

Design features: this includes layout of rooms, size, attractiveness and colour schemes.

Single bedrooms: providing opportunities for:

- personal space and territory
- privacy and freedom
- personalising rooms
- retention of personal belongings
- somewhere to entertain.

Finally, a residence should always be kept in good condition and all damage and general repairs carried out with the same sense of urgency as would be the case in one's own home.

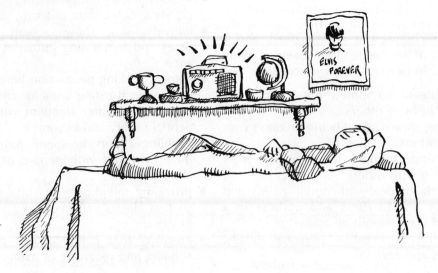

A SETTING IN WHICH TO GROW

The nature of the residential environment is significant in determining the extent to which growth and development can take place. An environment which focuses on client growth is based on:

The notion of dignity of risk
Democratic or shared living.

Dignity of risk

The idea of dignity of risk is closely allied to the principle of normalisation. It suggests that personal disability should not prevent individuals from being in situations and encountering experiences which may be a potential or actual threat or risk to their well-being. It stands in opposition to beliefs of the past suggesting disabled people to be so physically and emotionally vulnerable or child-like that staff should protect them from experiences with a potential to harm. Where staff have taken such a protective role, the result has been to smother, restrict, inhibit and control client lives.

Risk is an essential aspect of life and development and it should not be denied to disabled people. It can become a reality in their lives by:

- allowing, encouraging and teaching them to do as much as possible for themselves
- enabling them to be on their own in situations of potential risk
- encouraging learning by trial and error rather than having everything so structured that failure can never occur
- developing involvement beyond the residence
- allowing them to experience, on both a social and emotional level, the positive and negative consequences of their behaviour
- not making aspects of the living environment abnormally protective. Apart from the obvious need for certain modifications providing access for physically disabled clients, aspects of the building which reduce risks, such as doors without locks and bath taps which clients cannot control, are often counter to the idea of dignity of risk.

Enabling clients to have greater responsibility and to experience risk situations also entails risks for staff in that they can be held to account for what happens to clients. It is therefore essential that there is:

- adequate understanding between all levels of helpers in the early stages of increasing the risk dimension in client lives, and reassurance that direct care staff will be supported should problems arise
- recognition that exposing clients to risk should be a gradual process. It is important to distinguish between situations where a slight risk may be involved and those where there is a distinct element of danger
- an appreciation of the differences between dignity of risk and neglect.

Democratic or shared living

Clients have a right and a need to be fully involved in decisions in their residence. It is therefore necessary to increase levels of participation to make decision-making more democratic.

That is not to suggest the immediate adoption of a decision-making process on the basis of a majority vote, although over certain matters that may be appropriate, but that there should be a much greater degree of shared decision-making in a residence, both informally in the context of everyday discussions and formally by holding regular meetings.

Democratic living involves continuous processes of negotiation both on formal and informal levels. It is a fact that groups of people living and working together naturally and legitimately have different goals, and disagreements among them are best resolved not by the exercise of authority but by negotiation. This means that clients and helpers should always be prepared to change their positions on issues to arrive at mutually acceptable standards and practices.

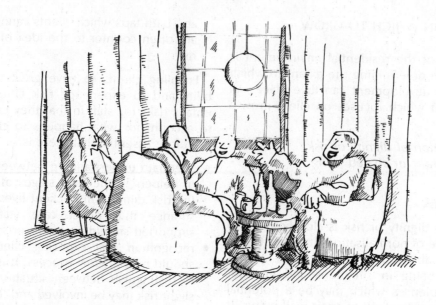

An environment that enables clients to be involved in decision-making processes is also one that leads to:

- greater consideration for and toleration of other people
- greater individual responsibility
- more open and frank expression of views, suggestions, complaints and grumbles
- closer, less cautious and more trusting relationships
- greater variations in lifestyle.

Increasing client involvement cannot become a reality unless helpers think and function in appropriate ways. This includes being able to:

- fully comprehend the needs of clients both individually and as a group
- initiate processes to bring about necessary changes in the pattern of daily life
- give up the power they have over clients and to operate without formal, non-negotiable rules
- tolerate, support and evenencorage disagreements
- operate without clear status barriers such as formal titles and uniforms or separate and superior dining facilities

- share daily life including recreation, domestic tasks, holidays and celebrations.

Increasing client involvement in decision-making can be brought about by encouraging client meetings and establishing client committees which, in larger facilities, should be recognised as representative and negotiating bodies. Staff involvement or participation in such meetings or committees should be by invitation.

In establishments where clients have been kept in a dependent state and have not been involved in decision-making, progress towards greater involvement may at first be difficult. Indeed, too rapid movement in this direction can create immense problems and actually be unfair to clients. It can, for example:

- lead clients to make quite unrealistic demands
- create immense hostility, both in clients and staff
- lead to the dominance of a group by one or two more manipulative members.

An effective way of increasing participation in decision-making is to begin by involving clients in relatively minor but nevertheless significant decisions, such as choice of food or television programs.

A SETTING FOR GREATER INDEPENDENCE

Clients have many personalised needs which, when met, contribute significantly to:

- the quality of their lives
- their self-concept
- their capacity for independent action
- their growth towards greater maturity
- acceptance of them by others

They have a right to these needs being recognised and effectively met and to exercise responsibility for them. The purpose of the discussion in this section is to suggest appropriate attitudes and standards so that clients can be helped to achieve greater independence. Among the more important needs are those relating to:

> *Clothing*
> *Personal hygiene*
> *Hair*
> *Personal possessions*
> *Money*
> *Food and dieting*
> *Smoking and alcohol.*

Clothing

Clothes are of considerable importance to most people. However inattentive they may seem about their dress, their clothes are part of their identity, serve as a statement as to how they wish to be perceived, and are significant in determining how others evaluate them. Wearing clothes that are personally chosen is a form of self-expression and contributes to a sense of personal dignity and self-esteem.

The standards and expectations used in relation to the clothes of disabled people will be the same as those for other people in society, that is, the clothes of clients should be:

- chosen by them
- their personal property and responsibility
- purchased specifically by them from shops in the community
- kept in their bedrooms or near their personal space in a lockable wardrobe or cupboard to which they have unrestricted access
- available for them to wear if they so choose

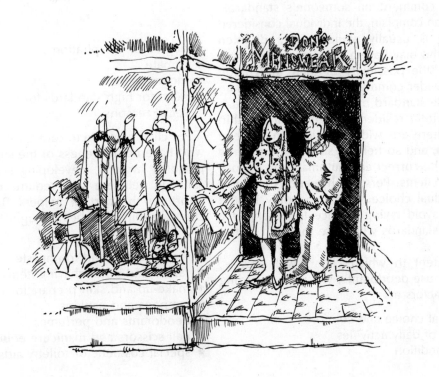

- identified by an inconspicuous and attractive name tag if there is a likelihood of them being misplaced.

Clients have a right to decide what clothing to buy and wear. It may at times be necessary to help them make choices so as to acquire skills to discriminate in terms of appropriateness and inappropriateness. Where, as a result of organisational factors or large numbers of clients, there may be problems in using shops in the community, these difficulties can be reduced by involving families and volunteers, or by asking individual members of staff, as key workers, to be involved in the purchase and general care of the clothes of one or two clients. Some clients may not appear to be concerned about what they wear. They should, nevertheless, have the opportunity and be encouraged to develop an interest in their clothes and having done so, sustain it if they so desire.

Personal hygiene

Personal hygiene is seen as an individual matter and, beyond the living group, it is not usual to comment on someone's standards. Rather than complain, the individual considered offensive is usually avoided. For disabled people who may have a problem in this area, there is little possibility of their integration into the wider community until they reach an acceptable standard of personal cleanliness.

Both within residential settings and within society there are wide variations in hygiene standards, and so helpers should not assume theirs to be correct and automatically impose them on clients. Personal hygiene is a matter of individual choice, influenced only by the need to avoid giving offence to others as a result of standards which are too high or too low.

The extent to which clients will shower, bathe, or use deodorants, will vary according to such factors as:

- personal choice and comfort
- nature of daily activities
- skin condition

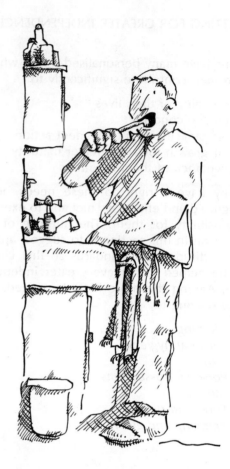

- degree of perspiration
- climate
- incontinence
- need for high standards for occupational or social reasons.

For clients unable to care for themselves, or who have no awareness of the significance of personal hygiene, developing standards and skills in self-care will require considerable effort on the part of helpers. This involves clients owning and being taught to use:

- soap and shampoo
- toothbrushes and toothpaste
- razors and other shaving items
- make-up and skin preparations
- tampons and napkins
- deodorants and perfumes
- nail scissors and manicure equipment
- special cosmetic or toiletry aids.

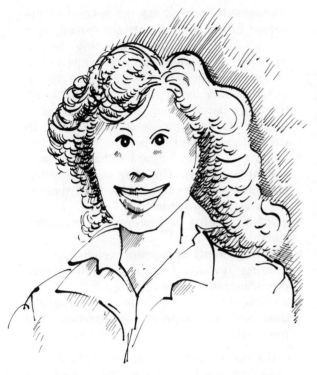

Hair

Hair, like clothing, is usually a significant aspect of an individual's self-identity. For many there is nothing so depressing as a hairstyle which makes them feel and look unattractive.

Improving standards of hair care for clients can be attained by:

- teaching them to wash and look after their hair
- advising them on what style suits them. This can be aided by making available magazines which illustrate differing styles
- enabling them to use hairdressers in the community
- allowing them to experiment with styles and follow fashion however outrageous it may appear to helpers.

Personal possessions

The congregate nature of many residential settings has made it difficult for clients to retain personal possessions. Life has been so open, public and impersonal that some clients, far from having a cupboard full of personal items, have never known what ownership means.

Personal possessions are highly significant dimensions of self, and if they have been given by someone of importance, have particular meaning. It is thus essential to provide environments which make it possible for clients to retain articles they value. This can be achieved by:

- encouraging them to bring possessions with them when they move into a residence
- teaching clients the meaning of ownership and the importance of respecting that which belongs to others
- making it necessary for them to own certain items such as soap, razor and clothes
- providing each client with a secure place to keep possessions
- ensuring that what is given to them is theirs and does not become communal property
- enabling them to learn what lending and sharing means
- enabling clients who would not otherwise have personal possessions to acquire them
- taking appropriate action when something belonging to a client has been stolen, including strong disapproval on an emotional level.

Money

Living normally involves having, being responsible for and spending money. It therefore follows that clients, like others, should have some form of income, however small, which is at their disposal. In ideal terms that income should be earned or be in the form of a pension or benefit out of which they would pay in their way, rather than the costs of their care being deducted without their involvement.

Whatever income clients receive, apart from that which they have worked for, inherited or have been given, should be based on an agreed and equitable scale. The payment of money to clients should be carried out in a decent and personalised way rather than in an institutional process. The term pocket money is perhaps best avoided for adults since it has child-like connotations and suggests gratuity.

While clients may reasonably be expected to purchase certain essential items for themselves, they should never be expected to buy that which should be provided for them. More importantly, their income should never be manipulated as a form of reward or punishment.

Teaching some clients to value and handle money is a process that may need to begin at a very elementary level by helping them to recognise coins and notes and their differing values. Once they have some awareness of what money means they should be permitted to experiment with its use, not merely as a learning experience but because they are entitled to do so. They should, therefore, have opportunities to spend or save their money. This will involve visiting banks, shops and places of interest and entertainment.

Food and dieting

As in the case in mainstream society, there are often problems of obesity in residential accommodation, and it is a rare establishment that does not forever have some clients on diets. While on health grounds and in relation to standards of attraction, overweight may be undesirable, decisions about what food and how much of it clients should eat will be theirs to make. Imposing a diet upon a person is an unacceptable practice, whatever the reason, and it is a violation of individual rights. Restricting food intake should be something a client freely agrees to. In any event, attempting to make people lose weight by imposing diets is seldom if ever successful because individuals can usually circumvent them and obtain all the food they want.

It is therefore important to approach the problem of overweight in a supportive and helpful way. This can be achieved by:

- attempting to discover the cause of the

problem. Its origins may be related to the nature of the food clients are served, or a liking for particularly fattening foods. Alternatively, a client may overeat as a form of compensation and a response to an unsatisfactory living situation. Perhaps, on the other hand, it may simply be related to a total lack of exercise, or being made to eat all food served on plates
- helping clients to be aware that they have weight problems. This may take considerable time and should be done in as supportive a way as possible
- involving clients in devising and preparing suitable diets
- teaching clients to monitor weight loss
- offering rewards for success rather than punishments for failure
- viewing diets as part of broader programs designed to improve appearance and personal care.

Reducing weight is just as difficult for disabled people as it is for others. Evidence indicates that most people on diets fail to lose a significant amount of weight or, if they do, the loss is rarely permanent. Successfully losing weight usually involves radical changes in attitudes towards self, food, eating habits and often in total lifestyle. Thus it is unlikely to be achieved merely by the imposition of a diet.

Smoking and alcohol

If clients are legally entitled to do so, they should not be prevented from smoking and drinking beer, wines or spirits merely because they live in a residential facility. To smoke and enjoy alcohol are seen as rights in society and a matter of individual choice. Since, however, clients live with others who may have quite different standards, practices relating to smoking and drinking may not simply be something for the individual to determine. Other factors to be taken into account will be:

- whether personal habits associated with smoking and drinking cause genuine offence to others

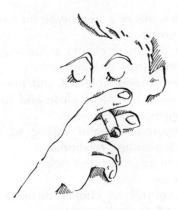

- whether smoking habits cause fire risks
- the effects of alcohol on behaviour.

In general, clients should be helped to learn that their own habits and preferences may need to be moderated out of respect and consideration for others.

Problems in relation to smoking can be dealt with by:

- agreeing on certain rooms for smoking
- provision of sufficient ashtrays
- teaching responsibility in the use of matches and disposal of cigarette butts
- dealing with specific difficulties as they arise rather than making general rules as a result of the single occurrence of an incident.

As far as alcohol is concerned, a most important factor to consider is whether alcohol and a client's medication are incompatible. Where this is the case and the medication is essential, the client should be informed of the consequences and advised not to drink.

Unless there are strong reasons to the contrary, alcoholic drinks should not be considered as being different from other beverages. In general, the use of alcohol in the context of social relationships and as a dimension of leisure is accepted and desired by most people. It therefore should be responsibly integrated into the pattern of life of a residential environment rather than be something which is covert. Perhaps this is best done initially on a group basis by purchasing drinks for special occasions and celebrations. Beyond that, what individuals do at other times, as long as they cause no major problems for others, is essentially their concern.

The issues of smoking and alcohol, like those of diets, physical contact and sexual behaviour, are areas where there are widely diverging standards in society. There will be staff and clients who feel that their personal standards should govern not only their own behaviour but that of others. It must be the case, however, whatever the intensity of personal convictions, that individuals should see themselves as having no right to impose their standards on others. As far as staff are concerned, whatever power they have should never be used to compel adult clients to behave according to their own or someone else's personal beliefs or moral standards.

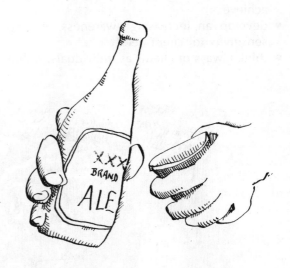

A SETTING FOR MEANINGFUL RELATIONSHIPS

Many of the more significant needs of human beings can be met only as a result of close and meaningful relationships. Residential settings for disabled people should be contexts where such relationships can be developed and maintained.

Close interpersonal relationships are usually characterised by:

- reciprocity
- intimacy
- spontaneity
- feeling and emotion
- caring and concern
- respect and significance
- difference and negotiation.

A residence should encourage the development of significant relationships between all members, that is, between groups of clients and groups of staff as well as between staff and clients. In regard to relationships between direct care workers and clients, there is much that helpers can do to establish and maintain them. They should, for example:

- operate from a positive personal philosophy about what they are attempting to achieve
- develop an increasing awareness of, and sensitivity to, client need
- think always of clients as individuals, rather than in terms of a stereotype for a particular client group
- learn to evaluate clients according to abilities rather than disabilities
- be warm, open, tolerant and non-authoritarian so as to enable close and supportive relationships to develop
- be prepared for, and willing to develop, more demanding relationships
- allow clients and other helpers freedom of expression
- avoid control of clients through punishment and reward systems
- converse with clients rather than restrict communication to directives; in other words, talking with rather than at or down to them
- apologise openly for mistakes
- strive generally to be good models in the area of relationships
- resist client ingratiation and humbling behaviour
- allow clients to choose the staff they wish to relate to and to determine the depth of relationships

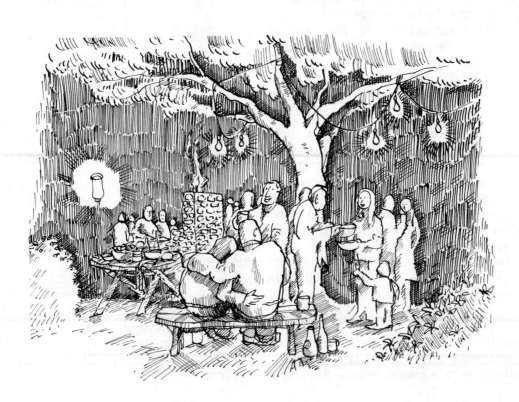

- try to prevent organisational pressures from reducing the quality of relationships.

Staff also have a role in fostering relationships among clients and with people beyond a residence. This they can do by:

- recognising the importance and significance of such relationships
- giving clients freedom to get to know others
- providing a reasonable context for the development of relationships
- enabling clients to choose those with whom they wish to live
- keeping groups of clients together and not moving individuals without consulting them and without good reason
- helping to resolve some of the problems clients experience in interpersonal relationships
- ensuring that important times of the day, such as meal times and leisure times, are conducive to the development of positive relationships
- welcoming clients' visitors
- teaching appropriate social behaviour associated with relationships.

Physical contact and touch

Close interpersonal relationships are usually characterised by physical contact and touch. People touch, hug, stroke and kiss one another as demonstrations of feelings. In the residential context this dimension has relevance for relationships between clients, clients and staff and, in some situations, it may be an appropriate dimension for relationships between staff members. Physical contact is an important aspect of relationships because it:

- is a natural and spontaneous expression of regard
- is symbolic of liking and affection
- provides pleasure.

Physical contact should be viewed as an essential dimension of personal relationships in residential settings, providing it is age appropriate and consistent with the nature of help being offered. There are, however, a number of difficulties associated with it which sometimes cause staff to exclude it entirely from their helping approaches. Among these difficulties are:

- feelings of repulsion about some clients because of their physical state or personal habits
- fear of over-reaction among clients, such as jealousy and demand for contact, when helpers use touch discriminately
- the tendency sometimes to misread innocent gestures and see them as having sexual meaning
- concern about critical reactions of colleagues and clients' relatives
- conflict between formal expectations of staff on the one hand and the intimate nature of close relationships on the other
- inconsistencies in the way helpers use physical contact and touch.

While these problems are real, they need to be faced if relationships are to become normal and helpful. Staff can attempt to deal with them by:

- recognising that physical contact and touch are integal to close relationships
- being aware of the impact of physical contact and touch on clients both individually and in the group context
- discussing openly problems as they arise
- assisting and supporting individual workers who may have difficulties in this aspect of relationships
- being aware of occasions and situations where demonstrable gestures are not appropriate or are capable of being misunderstood
- enabling clients to become more attractive and touchable
- teaching clients appropriate expression of feeling.

Sexual issues

It is recognised today that the sexual desires

and needs of disabled people are no different from those of other people. The rules and conventions that apply to their behaviour should, therefore, be the same as those prevailing in the wider society. This means that clients have the right to behave according to their own standards irrespective of the beliefs of staff, or the extent to which they are aware of the meaning or moral consequences of what they do. The only formal limitations that should exist will be related to behaviour that violates the criminal code, exploits others, is cruel or abusive, or is too public.

To argue thus is not to advocate a totally *laissez-faire* approach or to impose sexual licence. Client limitations in knowledge, capability, experience and responsibility make it essential that staff provide a pattern of life and learning which will enable clients to act appropriately, to make choices and exercise discretion.

If clients are to have opportunities for enjoying the sexual aspects of relationships, the following areas should be considered:

> *Beliefs of helpers*
> *Recognition by helpers of the normality of sexual interest, exploration, excitement and behaviour*
> *Recognition of problems disabled people may have faced in their development*
> *Sex education*
> *Greater opportunities for normal social interaction*
> *Special help for certain physically disabled people*
> *Reducing the public nature of residential care.*

Beliefs of helpers

It may be necessary for helpers to critically question their beliefs concerning sexuality and sexual behaviour in order to be aware of the base from which they operate. Where helpers have moral codes which are extreme in comparison with mainstream values, be they strict or permissive, they should recognise them for what they are and actively avoid imposing them on clients.

There is also a need for groups of workers to talk openly and frankly about this subject so that a consistent set of beliefs and approaches in relation to client behaviour can be developed.

Normality of sexual interest, exploration, excitement and behaviour

The interest of disabled people in personal and interpersonal sexuality should be seen as quite normal. There may be some disabled people, however, and possibly the more severely intellectually disabled who, while having normal drives, will not be aware of the impact and consequences of their actions or be able to protect themselves from exploitation. It will be natural for helpers to be more concerned about the behaviour of these clients and to ensure that their experiences are not exploitative or grossly abnormal.

Problems disabled people may have faced in their development

Past treatment of disabled people has meant that many have grown up witout acquiring adequate knowledge, having had normal experiences or having developed any personal identity in areas relating to sexuality. For example:

- if they have been raised in an institutional environment they may have:
  — witnessed open and abnormal displays of sexuality on which they may have modelled their own behaviour
  — lived for the whole of their lives with people of their own sex
  — never experienced close relationships between adults, so being denied an essential modelling process
  — never interacted normally with children and adolescents who were not disabled had very limited opportunities for childhood and adolescent sexual exploration
  — accepted staff beliefs that sex was not for them

— been exploited sexually and have come to regard it as normal
- if they have been raised at home they may have:
  — been totally isolated for most of the time from interaction with others in their own age group
  — never received any advice and instruction in the area of sexuality.

Sex education

The purpose of sex education is to enable clients to acquire sufficient knowledge and appropriate attitudes and values to be able to deal with their own sexuality, to relate appropriately to others and to initiate and sustain pleasurable sexual experiences.

Among the areas where there is a need for some kind of instruction, be it formal or informal, are:

- differences between sexes and male and female sexual maturity
- development of sex drives
- masturbation
- sexual intercourse
- homosexuality
- contraception and abortion
- pregnancy and birth
- responsibility in relationships
- initiating sexual encounters and relating sexually

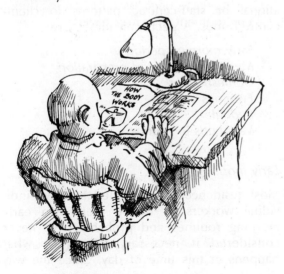

- developing relationships
- marriage
- laws about sexual behaviour
- genetic counselling.

Greater opportunities for normal social interaction

This will involve:

- seeking to eliminate congregate residences accommodating people of the same sex
- enabling clients to mix in the wider community
- providing them with opportunities to make friends and develop relationships
- reducing protective staff attitudes and practices.

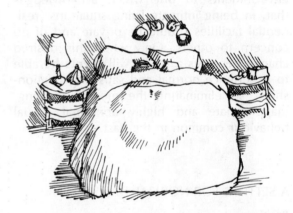

The most significant change that provides greater oppotunities for increased sexual freedom is the provision of single bedrooms. Once they are made available the question of appropriate and inappropriateness will be resolved by the simple fact of the ignorance of staff and others of client behaviour.

Specialised help for physically disabled people

Where clients have physical disabilities that prevent them from initiating or experiencing normal sexual encounters, they may need specialised help. This can involved:

- counselling

- provision of aids and instruction in their use
- direct involvement of a helper in enabling clients to enjoy each other sexuality.

Reducing the public nature of residential life

The influence of administrators, senior government officials and parents in many matters relating to residential care, together with the public nature of residential life, have contributed to sexual abnormality by creating considerable fear in staff about the consequences of allowing normal sexual freedoms.

It is now recognised that there is a need for a totally new approach in this area, from one based on the assumption that outsiders have the right to know what happens in residential environments to one which acknowledges that, in being intimate living situations, residential facilities should be private and of no concern to others. Only when this desired change becomes a reality will clients be able to experience normal and satisfying relationships, so eliminating the more disturbing, inappropriate and highly abnormal sexual behaviour common in the past.

A SETTING FOR NORMAL DAILY LIFE

Routines

There is a tendency today, because of the abnormality and rigidity of institutional patterns of life, to view routines as harmful to clients. While this view is understandable, it is, at the same time, important to acknowledge that routines are necessary because they:

- help a group maintain stability, order and continuity
- make life for individuals less confusing and more predictable and manageable
- provide a sense of security
- structure daily life.

At the same time, criticisms of routines in residential contexts can be justified where routines:

- are imposed without considering the real needs of clients
- are clearly in the interests of staff and are structured to minimise workloads
- are so rigid and ritualised that they stifle individual responsibility and initiative
- are inconsistent and chaotic because individual helpers create and impose their own routines in idiosyncratic ways
- structure the entire day
- bear no resemblance to normal life.

A reasonable routine in any residential environment will:

- be flexible
- be normalised
- be structured to reflect client need
- enhance client worker relationships
- minimise staff control
- be kept to a minimum, so enabling clients to act independently in many areas of their daily lives without direction from others
- be open to question and negotiation
- be understood, appreciated, agreed to and followed by both clients and staff.

Aspects of daily life

The remainder of this section considers the more important aspects of daily life with the goal of suggesting ways in which larger, congregate facilities can move from organisational or staff-centred patterns to client-centred ones. Aspects considered are:

Early morning period
Mealtimes and food preparation
Domestic work
Evenings
Bedtime
Variations in routine.

Early morning period

Most residences have tended to leave individual workers to devise their own early morning routines and probably have never considered it necessary to review what happens at this time of day. Since the way

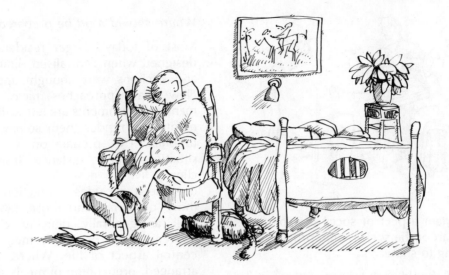

people are treated at this time can affect their whole day, and since there can be considerable inconsistency amongst staff, it is important to give attention to this period.

Among the issues to be considered are:

Is it necessary for staff to wake all clients?

Many can, in fact, be responsible for getting themselves up and staff should avoid sustaining unnecessary dependence.

What time should clients be woken?

An appropriate time will be determined in relation to:

- the age of clients
- the amount of sleep they have had
- reasons for getting up.

In general, the time of waking should be related to a client's first major commitment of the day, for example, attending school or work.

How should clients be woken?

Clients should be woken in a humane, considerate and personalised manner. Thus institutional practices such as ringing bells and shouting are not desirable. Clients should be approached individually, quietly called, given ample time to

wake, and not be expected to get out of bed immediately. For many, a second or third call may be necessary.

What should happen once clients are out of bed?

Once again this will vary according to many factors such as:

- conditions of clients on waking
- major commitments of the day
- amount of time available.

The issue of whether clients should or should not bathe or shower in the morning is essentially a problem to be resolved on an individual basis rather than according to some common standard and expectation.

Whatever happens at this time of day, there should not be an extended time period between getting up and having breakfast.

Meals

Mealtimes are not simply occasions for individuals to consume food but are essentially:

- social occasions with much symbolic and emotional meaning
- a way of enjoying the company of others

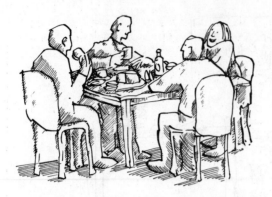

- an important aspect of social life, particularly as part of the socialisation process and in learning to share.

Thus staff should seek to ensure that mealtimes are pleasant and relaxed occasions. The more relevant questions to ask about mealtimes are:

What time should meals be taken?

There can, of course, be no one correct time. Timing for meals should be related to:

- client choice
- daily life of clients
- the times of other meals
- appropriate spacing of meals throughout the day.

The hours of work of staff, particularly those employed in kitchens, should not be a prior consideration and the major factor determining the times of main meals.

Where should meals be eaten?

Clients should normally have their meals in the part of the residence in which they live and with staff working there. Large dining rooms should, wherever possible, be avoided. Where it is quite impossible for meals to be taken in living units, partitioning a larger dining room so that smaller groups can eat together may be a short term solution. Only in exceptional circumstances should clients eat meals in bedrooms.

Where should food be prepared?

Most of today's larger residences were designed when centralised dining rooms and kitchens were thought appropriate. Now that approaches have changed, many establishments are left with arrangements that render them somewhat institutional. The preparation of food in situations some distance from where clients live is now seen as abnormal because it excludes interaction between those preparing and those eating it, as well as generally denying clients an awareness of, or involvement in, this central aspect of life. Where it can be arranged, preparation of meals should no longer take place in central kitchens but in individual living units. If this is not possible, a way of bringing about some improvemnt is to prepare meals in a central kitchen and take them in heated trolleys to living units. When there, they can be plugged in and the food kept hot until clients and staff wish to eat.

What choice of food should clients have?

At breakfast clients should be able to choose from a range of fruit juices, cereals and cooked dishes. It should be normal for them to help themselves and assist one another. Where it is not possible for clients to have a choice of dishes at the two major meals of the day, they should be involved in menu planning. A regular meeting where clients, direct care workers and kitchen staff meet to plan menus has many benefits, not least to cooks who get to know for whom they are preparing meals and what are the more popular dishes.

One obvious way in which clients express preference is by leaving food they dislike, and meals that prove to be unpopular should be removed from the menu. There is perhaps nothing more institutional than the same dish being served regularly yet seldom enjoyed. While there may occasionally be problems over client choice, such as unbalanced diet or monotony, such problems should not be viewed as providing sufficient reason for the control of menu planning by helpers. Creative cooking can often mean that food previously found unpalatable is now greatly enjoyed, and thus variation and balance maintained.

Finally, clients should be able to exercise choice over quantities served on their plates and how much they eat. Staff should never attempt to compel them to take or eat food they do not want.

How important is a balanced diet?

The issue of a balanced diet for clients seems a major problem for many workers. Whatever the feelings of helpers, whether or not clients keep to a balanced diet is largely a matter for them to decide. The task of helpers is not to impose their own standards but to educate clients so that they are able to exercise choice, control and responsibility over the food they eat.

Should food be used as reward or punishment?

The short answer to this question is in the negative. Food is a basic right, and not something to be given when clients please staff or to be denied when they do not. The insecurity and anxiety that is created when food is used as a form of manipulation is dehumanising. There may be some justification for withholding a less important but tastier course of a meal, such as a dessert, if children are being difficult at a mealtime or if their behaviour is an obvious form of resistance or confrontation. But this happens less frequently than helpers are sometimes inclined to believe, and where it does, it is equally likely that the staff involved are the major cause of the difficulty.

What about table manners?

Most people seem to have two sets of table manners, one for informal meals in the privacy of their homes and another for formal meals, either when entertaining guests, eating in restaurants or being entertained. If these are the normal standards in society then they are appropriate for residential care. Thus, breakfast in particular, which is the most informal meal of the day, should not be regulated by formalised table manners. For other meals, the practices of clients should not be questioned by staff so long as they do not give offence to others.

What should staff be doing?

As far as breakfast is concerned, if it is an informal meal and clients are coming and going, staff may well be involved in the

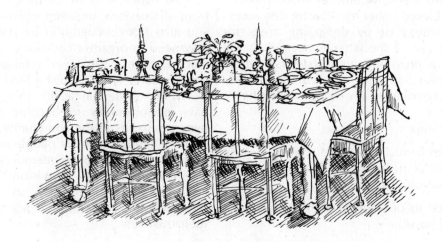

preparation of food or other related tasks. Where this is not the case, the most obvious and appropriate place, for breakfast as for other meals, is to eat with clients. One significant benefit when staff and clients share the same meal is that food is generally of a high standard. In addition, not only are helpers able to act as models for appropriate behaviour, they have greater chance of creating relaxed and enjoyable social situations which can be generalised to other aspects of daily life.

What about formal and informal meals?

As is the case with people in their own homes, there should be a mix between informal, everyday and quite formal meals. Informal meals will be those where clients come and go during the hours the meal is available, those taken while watching television and also picnics and barbecues. Formal meals will be those for special occasions such as birthdays or some other celebration. On such occasions, different kinds of food may be served and tables elaborately prepared.

Should clients be involved in food preparation?

Where clients are able to make their own meals and be involved in the preparation of food, they should be expected to do so. Additionally, they should also be able to have snacks when they wish. This can be achieved either by allowing free access to kitchens or by equipping areas for client use. If the latter is desired, it will involve providing jugs, toasters, cutlery and also supplying tea, coffee, biscuits and ingredients for making sandwiches.

Domestic work

In many residential facilities clients are heavily involved in domestic work. This practice has come about because of:

- the need to operate facilities as inexpensively as possible
- the need to occupy clients
- the belief that domestic work was a form of treatment or therapy.

Much criticism has been made of this practice in recent years, not only because it can be a form of exploitation, but because client skills in domestic tasks have actually served as reasons for continued institutional care. It is of considerable importance to realise that clients are not a ready supply of cheap labour and that their use solely to maintain a residence is no longer acceptable. If clients wish to continue to work virtually full-time on domestic or maintenance tasks, staff should ensure that they are not being exploited and that they receive appropriate payment.

What tasks, then, can clients undertake? If they are living in small groups, they will share responsibility for daily chores with five or six other people, and so what they will do will not be for large numbers who are, for the most part, strangers to them.

Evenings

The period between conclusion of the evening meal and bedtime has traditionally been one of considerable difficulty in residential care. The goal for this time of the day should be to achieve a balance between leaving clients to do whatever they wish and organising them for the whole period.

What happens in the evening should result from discussions between clients and staff, and also from recognition by staff that they may need to organise constructive and enjoyable activities. Whatever arrangements are made, clients should not be limited to activities in the residential facility since they should have opportunities to become involved in leisure pursuits in the community.

The evenings of many people in residential settings, like most other members of society, are dominated by television, and it is important for staff to think about the way television is used where clients do not have their own sets.

In general:

- television should not be used as the only form of evening activity
- clients should choose the programs they watch unless there are particularly strong reasons to the contrary, as may be the case with children
- clients should never be obliged to watch television when they do not wish to
- a television should be positioned in a way that makes viewing pleasant and enables clients to control it.

Bedtime

Among the questions that may need to be considered are:

What time should clients go to bed?

Once again the answer to a question of this kind will be related to many factors such as:

- the ages of clients
- the time they have to get up
- how tired they are
- how much sleep they need.

Thus bedtimes will be established in relation to the needs of individual clients, and generally determined by them.

Should there be any rules about what clients wear in bed?

Unless there are strong reasons to the contrary, this is a question for clients to determine as, of course, is the question about the number of covers on the bed.

What should staff be doing at this time?

Some clients may need assistance with undressing or with other aspects relating to preparation for bed. Staff generally should seek to avoid behaving in inappropriate ways at this time and avoid over-involvement where it is not necessary.

When clients are asleep, they should be permitted to sleep without disturbance. Lighting should be reduced to a minimum, domestic noise and conversation kept down, and there should be no unreasonable practices in regard to the provision of fresh air and ensuring that all is well.

Variations in daily life

Whatever pattern of daily life is established, there will always be variations both for individuals and groups particularly:

- at weekends
- on public holidays
- for special occasions, for example, birthdays and other celebrations
- when clients have visitors
- at holiday times.

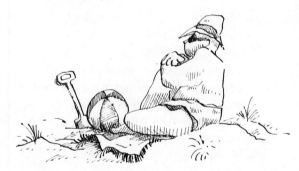

11

Developing small community residences

Small community residences are ordinary houses in the community in which disabled people live. They are a recent innovation in service provision and are likely to play an increasingly significant part in meeting the accommodation needs of disabled people. This chapter looks at reasons favouring the setting up of such facilities and the many factors to consider when developing and operating them.

WHY DEVELOP SUCH FACILITIES?

Small community residences are considered highly desirable because they:

- *provide a normalised context for meeting need.*
  Small residences are able to provide maximum opportunities for normal functioning because, in being like the residences of other people in society, they lend themselves to a similar pattern of life.
- *are consistent with the rights of disabled people.*
  Disabled people, irrespective of disability or social competence, have a right to live like other members of society, that is, within the community. This right to live within the community is, for most clients, consistent with their needs as defined by the principle of least restrictive alternative.
- *encourage the integration of disabled people into society.*

If disabled people live in a way that is no different from others, there is every likelihood that present perceptions of them as abnormal will diminish. Not only will this increase their integration into society, but it will make it impossible to discriminate against them on the grounds that, in living in special accommodation associated with deviant groups, they must themselves be deviant.

- *provide considerable opportunities for growth and development.*

The developmental approach asserts that growth towards maturity can only take place when individuals live in settings which place considerable and continuous demands on them. The small community residence has the greatest potential to provide such experiences because it necessitates a lifestyle which involves interdependence and obligation.

- *provide a home-like living context.*

Small residences have the greatest chance of being perceived by disabled people in need of residential assistance as their own homes. Such facilities offer all the social and psychological advantages associated with home; for example, maximum possibilities for security, privacy and intimacy; for individualising and personalising daily life and, above all, for developing a strong sense of belonging and attachment.

- *have already proven to be successful.*

Organisations in various parts of the world operating small community residences report immense changes in clients previously living in the more traditional forms of care, particularly those believed to be severely disabled. Evidence indicates that once clients have settled in new environments, they develop a wide range of skills and are able to exercise considerable responsibility. Furthermore, the obvious benefits of their new way of life enhances their self-concept and sense of worth.

Evidence indicates also that positive effects can be as marked for direct care workers in small community residences. This appears to have a great deal to do with the degree of autonomy that accompanies their new role. It is also a consequence of the absence of many of the more counterproductive forces common in the larger facility. Workers in community residences report immense job satisfaction and appear to have a high commitment to clients. The benefits they derive from this work situation generates supportive colleague relationships which in turn help to create a positive organisational climate.

In summary, then, the broad argument about small community residences is not whether they should be available to disabled

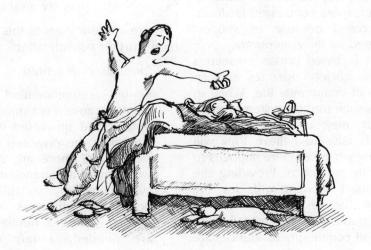

people; since such residences are obviously so beneficial, the focus should be on removing organisational and other barriers preventing their development.

Community residences: dubious justifications

Some arguments used to support the development of small community residences are highly questionable. To enable service providers and others to be clear about why this form of residence is favoured and to avoid justifying its introduction on dubious grounds, it is worth pausing to identify what these arguments are.

- *Small group residences are not as expensive as larger facilities.*
  Evidence in support has generally been limited to a calculation of the costs to an organisation of the actual provision of residences and the salaries of direct care workers. A realistic estimate must also include the cost of support services necessary to make them viable. When this happens they appear no less expensive than other forms of residential accommodation.
- *They are easier to organise and administer than are larger facilities.*
  The demands such resources place on organisations and staff are considerable. An effective system of community residences is likely to require far greater skills and abilities than are needed for the administration of larger, more centralised facilities.
- *They will succeed because of support systems provided by the community.*
  This argument is based on an erroneous notion of how society operates and an idealised view of community life. While in some localities such support systems can be developed, or may even occur spontaneously, it is false to believe they will come into being wherever there happens to be a community residence. Providing the necessary support services will, for the most part, be the responsibility of the organisation establishing the residence. In this sense, small community residences are

about assisting disabled people in the community, rather than by the community.

ESTABLISHING COMMUNITY RESIDENCES

Small community residences not only involve a different pattern of life for disabled people than is the case with other forms of residential accommodation, they necessitate different organisational structures and modes of operation.

Among the more significant factors to consider prior to establishing them are:

> *What exactly is a small community residence?*
> *The siting of residences*
> *Suitable forms of accommodation*
> *Support services*
> *Possible community reactions*
> *Family involvement*
> *Appropriate organisational structures*
> *Staffing factors*
> *Client factors*
> *Financial implications*
> *The pattern of daily living.*

What is a small community residence?

A small community residence is:

> *a purchased or rented house or flat in the community in which a group of probably not more than six disabled people live.*

There are four parts to this statement which merit further consideration:

> *'purchased or rented . . .'*

Rented accommodation is favoured by many because it is simpler and quicker to obtain, and unwanted houses can, at a later date, be disposed of easily. At the same time, there are certain problems with rented accommodation, such as the availability of suitable homes and occasional difficulties with owners or agents. Where a number of residences are needed, a mix of rented and purchased accommodation is probably the best arrangement. Some houses purchased by organisations can be let to groups of clients to give them a greater degree of independence.

'in the community . . .'

Homes used as residences should be no different from others in the neighbourhood and so will have no features, such as displayed formal names, unusual architecture or extended car parks, to set them apart and stigmatise clients.

Residences should be widely dispersed in the community so as to avoid particular districts having disproportionate numbers of disabled people which may attract unfavourable comment, hostility and abnormal treatment.

'not more than six disabled people . . .'

Because of limitations that may be imposed on lifestyles and also because of possible negative reactions of those living nearby, it is essential to ensure that groups of disabled people living in residences are not conspicuously larger than is normal in the neighbourhood.

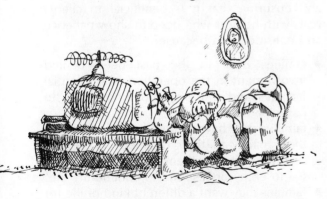

'disabled people live . . .'

A residence is essentially the home of those living within it and so outsiders, including helpers, should be seen as visitors with no natural right of entry. Staff who have keys should not normally let themselves in unless clients request it or it is necessary to do so.

The siting of residences

The siting of residences is an important consideration. Among the factors to be taken into account are:

- *proximity to services.*
  Residences should be near public transport, shops, banks, entertainment and day centres used by clients.
- *kind of neighbourhood.*
  The class of a neighbourhood should be appropriate to the clients, thus not so high or low as to be abnormal or to create problems. There have been suggestions that community residences succeed in areas where there is considerable movement of population because there is no stable community that can react in a hostile way.
- *location in a neighbourhood.*
  It is helpful for a residence to be fairly central in a neighbourhood so as to maximise possibilities for integration.
- *areas to be avoided.*
  The use of accommodation in business or industrial districts is not seen as particularly helpful because it provides no community into which clients can become integrated.
- *reality factors.*
  It may well be the case that the ideal types of residence are not available. Where this is so, it is probably better for clients to move into less than ideal forms of accommodation rather than wait for an indefinite period, hoping something more suitable will eventually be found.

Suitable forms of accommodation

Most homes available for rental or purchase will probably be suitable. There is no reason why the choice of building and its location should be related to the disabilities of clients unless, of course, they have certain physical disabilities.

When looking for suitable accommodation the following questions are worth asking:

- Is the house large enough for the group in question?

- What will it cost to rent and maintain?
- Is it physically integrated into the community?
- Is it close to public transport, shops, employment or day care facilities?
- Are there sufficient bedrooms for the clients to have rooms of their own should they so desire?
- Does it provide clients and neighbours with sufficient privacy?
- Is it in a reasonable state of decoration?
- Will it require a disproportionate effort to make it habitable?
- Is it sufficiently robust to stand knocks from clients not used to living in such confined spaces?
- If it does not have a telephone, are there any problems in having one installed before the residence is occupied?
- Does it have a garden which is not too small but which does not require upkeep beyond the capabilities of staff and clients?
- Are pets allowed?
- Is there a secure lease?

Support services

Clients in community residences are likely to require a range of services and other forms of assistance that should be provided either within the residence, brought to it or made available outside it. Among the more important services clients may need are:

- counselling and support
- laundry service
- housekeeper/homekaker
- personalised help and personal attendants
- home nursing
- home-based programs
- transport
- employment or other daytime occupation
- rehabilitation services
- leisure activities.

Possible community reactions

The success of community residences may depend upon the tolerance, acceptance and perhaps also the active support of neighbours. Experience in setting them up, however, suggests that unhelpful attitudes and unwarranted problems can be engendered where workers are overactive in informing neighbours about the use of accommodation and in soliciting support. It appears better to take a low key approach by occupying a residence without a great deal of ceremony, and responding to any difficulties that may subsequently arise. For the most part, opposition from neighbours has not proven to be a common problem. Quite often, within a short period of time, resistance and initial feelings of insecurity have given way to close and supportive actions. This does not mean, however, that neighbours and others do not experience problems and make complaints: they do, and this is an issue that is dealt with later in the chapter.

Family involvement

Where possible and appropriate, families should be encouraged to be involved in all phases of planning a particular residence and in supporting it once it is in operation. Responsibility for obtaining their involvement and ensuring that it is beneficial to clients rests with helpers who need to show patience and consideration because:

- families have in the past been denied involvement in the operation of residential facilities and thus may not know how to participate effectively
- families may have tended to underestimate the capacity of their disabled children or relatives and view them as having no potential to enjoy or respond to community life
- families may want a different kind of life for clients, such as a sheltered, protective environment, because of what they have been encouraged to see as appropriate by previous generations of helpers.

Family involvement can take place in many ways, for example:

- assisting in finding suitable accommodation

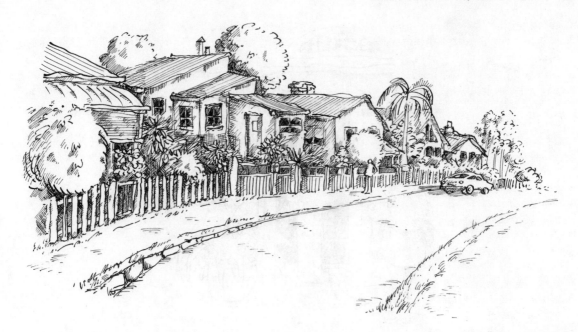

- obtaining items of furniture or domestic equipment
- sharing expenses
- preparing a residence for occupation
- visiting on a regular basis to assist with special tasks
- taking residents to outside daytime and leisure activities.

Appropriate organisational structures

Organisations seeking to establish community residences will need to develop appropriate philosophies and managerial systems. Essentially this entails:

- recognition that considerable organisational change is likely to be necessary to establish and effectively operate small community residences
- the transfer of resources from one service area to another
- loose and flexible ways of managing direct care staff with emphasis on support rather than control
- delegation of considerable responsibility and discretion to direct care workers
- programs of support and training for

members of staff who may not favour the idea of small community residences or who need additional skills to work in them effectively

- an approach which avoids judgments when things go wrong but which focuses on the problem-solving to put things right.

Staffing factors

The qualities and skills required of staff working in community residences will differ markedly from those of their counterparts in congregate forms of care. These differences will be most noticeable in relation to their:

Basic role
Hours of work
Special knowledge and skills.

Basic role

The small community residence is essentially the home of clients where workers are not expected to provide constant care but appropriate relationships and clearly identified services. When they visit, and sometimes this may be by appointment, what they do is likely

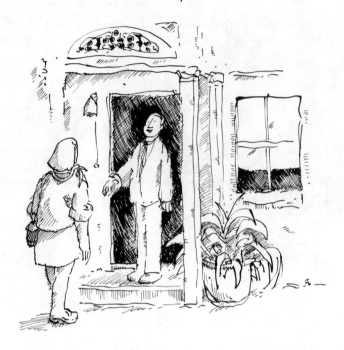

to be related to the reasons for their presence such as providing a specific service. Thus, they should not view themselves in parenting type roles.

The goal for staff is to help clients develop skills to enable them to live as independently as possible. Once clients begin to develop such skills the involvement of helpers should be reduced and their focus of attention change.

In addition to providing personalised services and relationships, helpers will have three other functions:

- to act as resource persons to enable clients to obtain services to which they are entitled
- to offer support to other people assisting or involved with clients, such as families, employers, volunteers, neighbours and community groups
- to act as advocates for clients.

Hours of work

Staff will not work in a residence according to the requirements of an inflexible and formally structured roster, but will be available in relation to client need. In a residence where serverely disabled people are living, for example, there may be a need for helpers to be present on a continuous basis; on the other hand, where clients are able to do much for themselves, a worker may only visit for a few hours each day or maintain contact by telephone. There will be occasions when staff will be required to assist clients during evenings and at weekends and so workers in community residences should not be those bound by a conventional sense of appropriate and inappropriate hours of work.

Special knowledge and skills

Effectively assisting clients in small community residences is likely to involve helpers in a number of fairly mundane but nevertheless important aspects of life. Not only is it necessary for helpers to acquire relevant knowledge and skills, they should seek to pass what they learn on to clients. Among such aspects are:

- knowledge of the social security system, for example, the range of benefits available to clients and how they can be obtained
- knowledge of various ways in which

housing can be obtained, that is, through real estate, housing commission, rental agencies, etc.

- knowledge of the legal system, including behaviour constituting civil or criminal offences
- knowledge of how to get clients included on the electoral role
- moving house, for example, removal arrangements, getting electricity and other services connected and disconnected, notifying others of new address
- medical arrangements, including general practitioners, dentists, ambulance services
- resources in the community which may be of benefit to clients
- domestic budgeting
- basic home maintenance, for example, changing light bulbs and fuses
- action to be taken in the event of emergencies such as severe illness, accident, intruders, fire and power failures.

Client factors

Among the factors to consider concerning clients and small community residences are:

> *General considerations affecting selection*
> *Actual process of selection*
> *Preparation.*

General considerations affecting selection

In a community residence clients will be living closely with a small number of others. It is essential that members of groups are selected carefully and on the basis of compatibility. Selection should be built around client choice and reflect the following characteristics:

- be based on a narrow age range, unless wide variation is by choice
- offer opportunities for living in a residence to both sexes
- reflect the mutual interests of clients
- seek to attain a balance of client skills and abilities.

Wherever possible, a group of clients living in a larger facility who appear to get on well, and wishing to do so, should move to a community residence together.

Actual process of selection

Since living in a community residence is a right and not something that should be earned, placement should not be limited by staff conditions or approval. Thus, places should not be offered:

- for good behaviour
- as a result of positive responses to preparation programs
- to those only having considerable social competence
- in the belief that a client's functioning will improve considerably as a result of community living.

In the early stages of developing community residences there are likely to be limitations both in the range and number of residences and in the availability of supporting services. This may be brought about by restrictions in finance, suitable homes or capable and willing helpers, and so it will be necessary to select those clients whose needs for community residence appear greatest. This can be achieved by:

- finding out which clients wish to live in such settings
- identifying those who have a realistic awareness of what would be involved
- identifying those who are adversely affected by their present residence, those, for example, who resent or do not benefit from the pattern of life it provides
- considering what specific behaviour or other problems are likely to make success in a community residence difficult for a particular client
- being aware of clients whose present behaviour would be disruptive to a small group living situation.

The following list of questions highlights some of the issues that should be explored at this stage:

- Has community living been discussed with the client?
- Does the client wish to live in a community residence?
- To what extent is the client aware of the way it is likely to change his/her life?
- Are there indications that the client's present living situation:
  — is not beneficial?
  — creates personal unhappiness?
  — is not the least restrictive alternative?
- Is the client likely to behave in ways which could adversely affect those he/she lives with or those living nearby? For example, is the client:
  — unreasonably noisy?
  — likely to dress inappropriately in or around a community residence?
  — aware that land and property belonging to others should not be intruded upon?
  — capable of behaving in a sexually appropriate manner?
  — likely to be physically or verbally abusive?
  — sufficiently honest for social living?
  — destructive to self or to property?

Preparation

Preparation for community living should not be seen as a prior condition for placement, not only for reasons suggested above, but because both the nature of the clients' present environment and their relationships with others may have created in them an inability to respond to preparation programs. Dependence on helpers, for example, or on parents, may have been so long standing that it is only when clients settle in entirely new environments that they are able to respond in positive ways and learn new skills. On the other hand, of course, some clients may never be capable of benefitting from preparation programs.

This is not to argue that preparation programs should not be attempted, for many clients they will be highly effective. The shape they take is likely to be dependent upon:

- the extent to which clients are able to understand what this change in lifestyle will mean
- their learning capabilities
- conditions in the living situation from which they are to move
- what they need to learn to function successfully in a community residence
- kinds of support services that will be available in the community residence
- staff skills in running such programs.

Among the topics that can be included in preparation programs are:

- standards of personal care
- behaviour appropriate in the community
- living with others
- shared household tasks and decision-making
- preparation of food
- budgeting and money management
- use of domestic appliances
- medication
- shopping
- relationships with neighbours
- illegal behaviour.

In ideal terms, the facility in which clients have been living prior to moving will have prepared them as a result of a normalised pattern of life. Where this has not been the case, a special unit could be established within a facility to simulate the pattern of daily living in a community residence so that clients can become more familiar with what is likely to be their new way of life, and perhaps develop necessary skills. They can also learn more about life in a community residence through visits.

Preparation programs should, wherever possible, be developed, organised and run by those direct care workers who will be involved with the clients once they have moved. This will maximise adjustment in the new context and enable continuity in supportive relationships.

Financial implications

Setting up a residence is likely to involve

substantial financial outlay and this fact should be considered before a house is obtained for a group. Cost will be incurred in such areas as:

- bond and rental advances
- purchase of domestic equipment and furniture
- installation charges for certain services such as phone and electricity
- modifications for physically disabled people and provision of aids.

If clients are expected to meet most, if not all, of these costs they should know beforehand so that they can accumulate or acquire sufficient capital. If, on the other hand, the organisation views itself responsible, it will need to make appropriate provision in its budget or find other ways of obtaining what is needed.

On a somewhat different level, consideration will need to be given to arrangements for:

- managing clients' money where they are unable to do so
- payment of rent, electricity, gas and phone bills.

Pattern of daily living

The pattern of daily living in a community residence should:

- seek to be comparable to that of most people in society
- reflect the needs of clients, both individually and as a group
- be flexible so as to enable change to take place whenever necessary
- not be governed by a series of formal rules.

SEQUENCE FOR SETTING UP A RESIDENCE

It may be of help to work through the following steps when planning a community residence:

1. Identify a group of clients who may wish to live in this form of residence.
2. Discuss with them the idea of moving to a community residence and what is likely to be involved.
3. Begin a preparation program when clients are ready.
4. Contact families, where appropriate, discuss

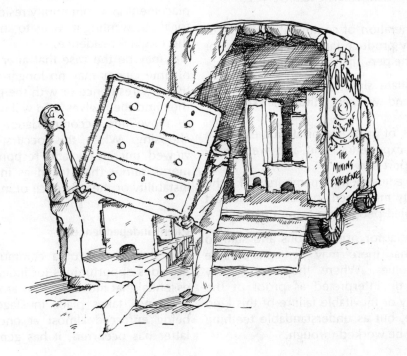

plans with them, get their support and, if possible, their involvement.

5. Seek suitable residences and involve clients in selection.
6. Estimate likely setting-up costs and ensure that sufficient finance is available.
7. Obtain furniture and furnishings and, with client involvement, carry out any necessary improvements, for example, alterations, redecorations, installation of telephone.
8. Determine initial staffing needs.
9. Determine initial support services such as:
   - day facilities
   - transport
   - recreation
   - services brought to the residence for individual clients or the group.
10. Organise removal.
11. Notify people and organisations of change of address.
12. Effect move.
13. House warming, inviting neighbours, staff, friends, families and others who may have contributed to setting up the residence.

OPERATING COMMUNITY RESIDENCES

The first generation of community residences will probably produce far more problems for clients and helpers than later ones because:

- they nessitate significant change in client lifestyle and worker attitudes, skills and behaviour
- of the lack of prior organisational expertise and staff experience, and also well-developed support services
- of the adjustment members of the community may need to make to the fact that disabled people are living nearby.

It is essential for organisations and staff to recognise that there may be considerable initial difficulties. Where they occur they should not be interpreted as proof of the undesirability or inevitable failure of this kind of residence, but as understandable teething problems to be worked through.

Among the problems and issues likely to be encountered are those relating to:

Client adjustment
Client independence
Financial limitations on client lifestyle
Occurrence of vacancies
Problems with neighbours
Illegal behaviour
Help from senior staff
Changes in support provided by direct care staff.

Client adjustment

The first groups moving to community residences are likely to have lived in congregate environments for many years. The pattern of life in the larger residential facility is usually quite different from that of the small community residence and clients may not be prepared for it. They may, for example, find their new life difficult and confusing and wish to return to the setting in which they had previously been living. Where they are clearly unhappy, a request to return to the original residence should be met. On the other hand, problems of this kind can be alleviated if placement in a community residence involves, for those wanting it, visits to and weekends in the original residence.

It may be the case that after a brief period of time clients may no longer wish to live in the new residence or with the group in which they find themselves, and will express a desire to move into accommodation of their own choosing. When this occurs it should be viewed uncritically and responded to on its merits rather than taken as indicating client instability or the existence of major problems.

Client independence

The style of life of a community residence provides opportunities for independence. It is essential that movement towards greater independence takes place in stages rather than being enforced almost at once. Where the latter has occurred, it has generally resulted in failure and a consequent retreat to controlling practices on the part of helpers.

Financial limitations on lifestyle

When clients become free from the impositions associated with an institutional lifestyle they often seek different patterns of life for themselves. A major limiting factor they can encounter is insufficient finance. Their incomes are usually quite low, and to avoid immense financial difficulties, debt or over-expectation about lifestyle, it is necessary to help them develop standards consistent with incomes. At the same time, where it is evident to helpers that clients have insufficient incomes or pensions they should press for increases by advocating on behalf of the clients.

Occurrence of vacancies

When individual clients move from a residence vacancies will be created. On the occasions this happens it is important not to consider a vacancy merely as an available bed to be filled at the earliest possible moment. It may be possible to leave it unfilled or to reduce the number of clients the residence is understood to accommodate if those remaining do not wish to have another person moving in, and if they are willing to meet any additional costs. Where the vacancy is to be filled, clients should be fully involved in the selection of the new member, and the final choice should normally be theirs.

Problems with neighbours

While problems with neighbours are not bound to occur, where they do they should be viewed as neither surprising nor unwarranted. Difficulties may arise because:

- neighbours may perceive a group of disabled people living nearby as threatening and feel genuinely concerned
- neighbours may have little understanding of or skills in relating to disabled people
- clients may behave in odd, disturbing or unacceptable ways because they have not yet learned behaviour appropriate to community living.

Complaints and difficulties should be treated seriously, even where they reflect considerable prejudice. When trying to resolve them it is important to:

- encourage complaints to be made to clients and direct care staff and not to organisations
- try to understand situations from the complainant's point of view
- work to resolve difficulties in ways that are acceptable to all and which reduce the chances of recurrence.

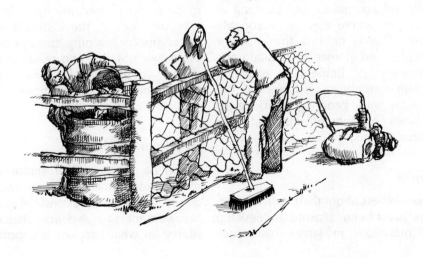

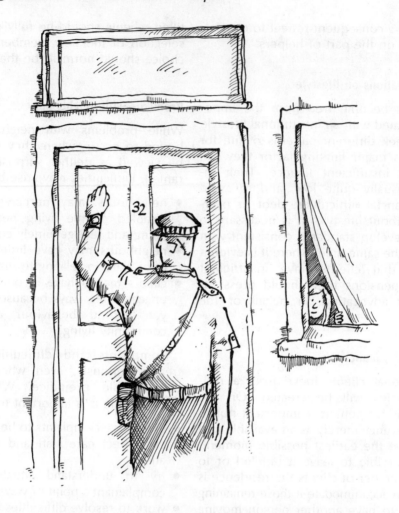

Being a neighbour involves recognising that those living next door are entitled to live as they so choose. This does not mean, however, total passivity and acceptance but working to achieve a situation where there is reasonable give and take. This is no less the case for disabled people, and it may necessitate the active involvement of helpers in resolving difficulties with neighbours, supporting the rights of clients and generally working to avoid the kinds of antagonisms that may otherwise develop.

Illegal behaviour

Because of past beliefs about their deficiencies, many clients have been allowed to develop patterns of behaviour in larger residences which, when displayed in the community, are offensive or illegal. Often clients and staff will not realise this until a complaint has been made or police become involved. When such episodes occur they should be seen as occasions for learning appropriate behaviour. Wherever possible and reasonable, therefore, clients should not be protected from the consequences of their actions.

Help from senior staff

It will be necessary for senior personnel or more experienced staff to support clients, direct care workers and residences. Their involvement and also acceptance of responsibility for what happens is important because:

- the risks associated with community residences can be considerable. Making certain decisions involving an element of risk will not be easy for direct care staff and should not be their sole responsibility.
- there are likely to be many problems which will need skilled input, for example:
  — complaints from clients about other clients, or from people outside a residence
  — changes in the life situation of one or more clients, such as illness or loss of employment
  — the behaviour of the majority of a group exploiting the minority and vice versa
  — individual clients getting into financial difficulties
  — inappropriate involvement of families
  — individual clients needing skilled counselling on specific issues, for example, family problems, sexual relationships, problems at work, recreation needs
  — the tendency for some helpers to be over-controlling
  — selection of clients to fill vacancies
  — difficulties associated with the direct care worker role in terms of isolation from colleagues and closeness to clients.

When direct care workers and clients develop skills to deal with these issues the involvement of more senior staff can be reduced.

Changes in worker support

It is likely that clients, once living in community residences, will achieve considerable competence in many areas of life. It follows, therefore, that when this occurs direct care staff involvement should be decreased. On the other hand, there may be occasions for an increase in staff attendance, at times of sickness, for example, or when a more able client leaves. Thus the support staff give to a residence should be seen as flexible and related to client need.

Helpers and families in partnership
Involving families
Problems with families

12

Family involvement in residential life

Since the focus of this book is on assisting disabled people in residential contexts, its content in relation to families is necessarily limited. This brief chapter seeks only to offer a range of ideas to enable helpers to involve families in residential life, and excludes consideration of a number of wider issues such as the way residential facilities can assist families caring for disabled people at home.

Contemporary approaches are built upon and stress the importance of the family, particularly for disabled children. Thus it is argued that:

- living within a family is, for most disabled children, the appropriate context for meeting their needs
- parents are as responsible for their disabled as their able children
- parents should be involved in all decisions that affect their disabled children
- many residential services should be viewed as forms of support for families caring for disabled children
- families should, wherever appropriate, be involved in the lives of relatives who live in residential accommodation
- families should be encouraged, supported and assisted by helpers so that they:
  - can relate on an equal basis with helpers
  - are able to question the quality of services provided
  - can establish and operate their own services and support groups

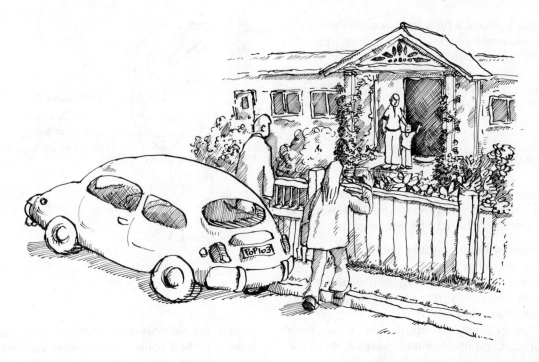

— can actively press, individually and collectively, for increased or improved services

— are able to play a significant part in the design, management and operation of residential facilities.

HELPERS AND FAMILIES IN PARTNERSHIP

The view today is that helpers, clients and families should work together in a manner that reflects the idea of partnership. In the context of helping relationships such partnerships will be characterised by equality, mutuality and sharing, with few status differences and no predetermined notions about superiority and inferiority.

Such partnerships will be possible when the following beliefs become integral to the philosophies of helpers:

- Generalisations about disabled people and their families are often unhelpful when seeking to identify and respond to individual need
- Parents should be accepted on their own terms, and theoretical perspectives which view them negatively should be seen as counter-productive
- Families are capable of knowing what help they require
- Families can be experts in relation to their own situation, and most have the potential to develop necessary helping skills
- Professional efforts are often of little value without family involvement
- Parents and relatives are able to make major contributions to the provision of services and the quality of life in residences
- Families have a right to full knowledge of the range of sevices available and how they can be obtained.

Effective partnerships between helpers, disabled people and their families are normally built upon such factors as:

- considerable patience and empathy on the part of helpers in order to understand a situation from the perspective of a family.
- the presence of parents or appropriate relatives at relevant decision-making conferences
- abolition of traditional conceptions of

confidentially which have meant the denial of essential information to clients, parents and appropriate relatives

- discretion in discussions with families so that comments made and views expressed are positive and helpful.

INVOLVING FAMILIES

Parents and close relatives should be encouraged to become fully involved in residential care settings. This can be achieved by:

- involving them in intake decisions and planning meetings
- providing them with literature about the goals and philosophy of a residence and its pattern of daily life
- helping them to appreciate what their support and involvement means both to the work of a residential facility and to their relative or child
- ensuring that all staff, and particularly direct care workers, recognise the value and importance of family involvement. This will mean creating in staff positive attitudes towards families and encouraging them to find the time to be available when parents and relatives visit
- encouraging families, where they are able, to maintain certain responsibilities for their disabled child or relative, such as:
  - provision and care of clothing
  - purchase of toiletries and hobby materials
  - transport to outside activities
  - provision of personal items such as radios, clocks and books
- encouraging frequent visiting at any time for as long as parents, relatives or clients wish, and with no restrictions on movement within a facility
- ensuring that the first visit in particular is a pleasant and successful one
- providing meals for parents and relatives who are interested in being involved in daily life
- providing meals or overnight accommo-

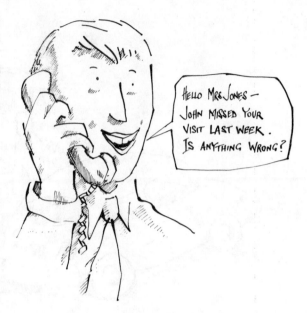

Hello Mrs Jones — John missed your visit last week. Is anything wrong?

dation for parents and relatives who may have travelled some considerable distance

- encouraging and enabling parents and relatives to become fully involved in the life of the residential setting. This may mean giving them some direction in what they can do to help
- arranging special events and celebrations to which parents can be invited
- involving parents in specific programs, not only as extra pairs of hands, but to enable them to acquire the necessary skills to continue such programs or operate similar ones during visits home or once the client has left the residence
- teaching parents to recognise growth and development when it takes place and, where necessary, encouraging them to alter their beliefs about the potential of clients
- involving parents in recreational and leisure activities
- being open and receptive to comments, criticisms and complaints from parents and taking all necessary action
- recording visits and make enquires of parents whose contacts have decreased
- involving parents and relatives in support groups and parent organisations
- encouraging parents to have clients home for evenings and weekends

- involving parents in major events affecting clients such as change of residence, sickness or accidents.

PROBLEMS WITH FAMILIES

If helpers are competent and professional in their dealings with families there is no reason why relationships should not be positive and beneficial. Occasionally, however, there may be difficulties. These are usually in the following areas:

- parents or relatives seeking to retain inappropriate control of adult disabled people
- parents or relatives wishing to dictate the

pattern of life, or caring, domestic or moral standards in a residence
- parents or relatives insisting on close involvement with clients when this is neither wanted by, nor helpful to, clients.

Where clients are adults, the involvement of parents and relatives should be governed by standards appropriate to society. If parents and relatives have unreasonable expectations, they should be helped in a way that enables them to understand, come to terms with and support approaches that are in the best interests of the client. Viewing parents in a hostile way and seeking to exclude them from involvement benefits no one, particularly clients.

13

Fostering community integration

One of the most important objectives of contemporary approaches is to achieve greater social integration of disabled people. While there are considerable possibilities of this occurring when clients live in small community residences, it may not be so for those living in larger and more isolated facilities. The aim of this chapter is, therefore, to offer ideas to enable helpers in the more traditional forms of residential care to increase client integration. These ideas are explored from two directions, that is, what can be done to:

> *Integrate clients into mainstream society*
> *Involve members of society in residential life.*

INTEGRATING CLIENTS

Integrating disabled people into mainstream society is justified on the grounds that it:

- is a right
- provides experiences essential for normal growth and development. Nothing has greater potential for developing abnormal behaviour than isolation from mainstream society
- enables many personal and social needs to be met that are denied in segregated and isolated residences
- Is essential for achieving appropriate levels of independence

- provides opportunities for interacting with people other than helpers and fellow clients
- is a way of slowly breaking down barriers and altering distorted perceptions of disabled people.

In some residential settings movement towards client integration into the full spectrum of social life is probably still in its infancy. Barriers from without and resistance from within are often considerable, and unless the more aware helpers take an active part in attempting to increase client integration change may never take place. It is, in fact, the responsibility of all helpers to do what they can to encourage, if not pressurise, the wider community to make space for its disabled citizens. In the interests both of disabled people themselves and the wider society, the task of helpers is to work towards changing society's beliefs and practices so that full participation and involvement of disabled people comes to be seen as normal.

In order to make integration a reality, helpers will need to be actively involved in society and in its community groups, working to change attitudes and behaviour. This involvement is likely to take place in four ways:

> *Reshaping traditional beliefs about disabled people.*
> Many of society's beliefs about disabled

people are inaccurate and unreasonable and helpers should, in their dealings with others, take an approach that demonstrates lack of support for negative or outwardly sympathetic but patronising attitudes. They should also resist any treatment of clients which implies difference from other members of society.

Resisting the idea that disabled people are suitable recipients of charity.
Meeting the needs of disabled people is a matter of rights and entitlement, not of charity. This is not to argue that donations and gifts towards the cost of services are no longer appropriate but that what is accepted is not accompanied by unrealistic expectations and does not have abnormal consequences. The gift of a vehicle, for example, is usually more than welcome, but it should not be emblazoned with details about who donated it to whom. Offers of help that are inconsistent with contemporary approaches should be declined with explanations of the reasons why and suggestions about more suitable ways of helping.

Using the media to advocate integration.
This can be achieved by seeking interviews with press and television, writing special articles, making television programs and films and initiating publicity campaigns.

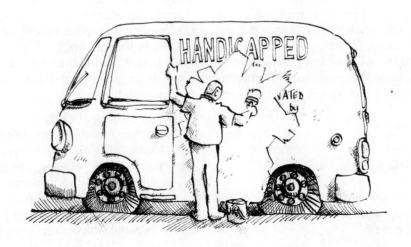

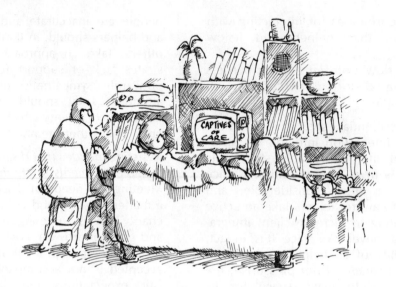

Responding to community problems involving disabled people.
Whenever difficulties occur, such as at school, at work, with neighbours or with police, helpers should seek appropriate involvement to ensure that the interests of clients are represented and safeguarded, and that others deal with them in normal ways.

A first step towards achieving greater integration will be the removal of restrictions on client movement. Where client involvement in the community has been a rare occurrence, helpers will need to actively involve them in a broad range of community-based activities. In order to reduce perceptions of abnormality, clients should rarely, if ever, go out in large groups; if they are to be integrated it will be in ones and twos. The days of mass outings and the crocodile of disabled people meandering its way along the main road, obstructing traffic or getting lost in shops, belong to the past.

INVOLVING THE COMMUNITY

There are two ways in which members of the wider community can become involved in the life of a residence:

As visitors
As volunteer helpers.

Visitors

Many members of the community, in addition to parents, relatives and friends of clients, have been frequent visitors to residential settings, for example:

- the general public on special occasions
- professional workers calling on clients or attending meetings
- church and other community groups for visits of interest
- students from schools, colleges and universities for visits of observation and work experience
- administrators from parent or other organisations for meetings
- politicians with interest in the resident group or who view visits as part of their responsibilities.

Visitors can be beneficial to a residential facility so long as the purpose of the visit and the actual visiting arrangements are consistent with the needs of clients, the pattern of life of a residence and the principle of normalisation. At the same time, the reality is that many residences remain part of large public or charitable organisations and criteria governing

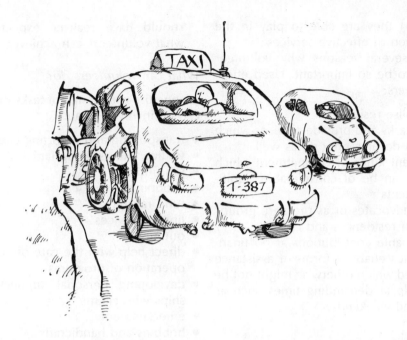

visits may continue to represent more organisational than client needs. Whatever considerations have to be taken into account, it is important to exercise proper control over this aspect of residential life and to realise that, in being the home of clients, certain limitations should be imposed upon all visitors. Visits certainly should not be permitted if the only reason is simply to come and stare.

There are a number of basic rules for ensuring that visits by those other than parents, relatives or close friends are beneficial:

- permission should be obtained from clients and direct care staff before visits are arranged
- groups of visitors should be scheduled for no more than one day each week
- a maximum number of visitors for any one group should be set and the number of people visiting known in advance
- information should be provided to visitors about what is expected of them, for example, rules for entering rooms and limitations on the use of cameras
- interactions between clients and visitors should be monitored when necessary to ensure that they are appropriate

- visitors should be offered adequate hospitality
- debriefing sessions should be held at the end of visits.

One form of visiting that has been very much part of the way of life of many residences is an outcome or holding fêtes or open days. While such occasions may have certain advantages in bringing outsiders into the establishment, gaining publicity and, perhaps more importantly, in raising money, there is little about them that is consistent with contemporary approaches and so they should be phased out.

Volunteers

A volunteer is:

> *an individual who offers time and skills to provide help that will, directly or indirectly benefit clients. No payment is made for what the volunteer does apart from reimbursement of certain minor expenses.*

The value of volunteers in residential situations is becoming increasingly recognised, and growth in their numbers reflects the significant part they are able to play in the overall provision of effective services.

There are several reasons why volunteer help is seen to be so important. Used effectively, volunteers:

- help normalise residences
- undertake tasks and provide services which staff cannot do or cannot do as well
- offer different kinds of commitment which sometimes can be of considerable significance to clients
- can act as advocates or as pressure groups on behalf of residences and clients
- make invaluable contributions at no financial cost, thus enabling forms of assistance to be offered which otherwise might not be
- provide help at demanding times such as evenings and weekends.

Volunteers: the reality

Volunteers clearly have a great deal to offer, and used effectively they can make the difference between an adequate and a good environment. At the same time it should be realised that:

- considerable time and effort is needed to recruit, select, train, deploy, support and retain volunteers
- the commitment of many volunteers will be short term. This should be seen as normal and in no way detracting from what they have to offer. Thus, there is likely to be a continual turnover of volunteers which should be accepted and expected.
- the quality of volunteer help is related to assistance, encouragement and support given by other helpers.
- the motivation and needs of volunteers should be understood, and where possible, matched by the tasks they are given.
- volunteer programs should not be started unless they can be maintained effectively. Poor programs are to be avoided since they affect the commitment and motivation of volunteers and have negative consequences for clients and staff
- many volunteers have limited skills. Staff responsible for or working with them

should have realistic expectations about what volunteers can achieve.

What can volunteers do?

Among the wide range of tasks that volunteers can be involved in are:

- transporting and escorting clients
- visiting and assisting families
- job finding
- shopping
- fund raising
- library services
- outings
- direct help with the care of clients and the operation of programs
- developing personal supportive relationships with clients
- entertainment
- hobbies and handicrafts
- educational tuition of children
- office work.

Whatever volunteers do, they should:

- not be viewed as a cheap form of labour
- not be seen merely as relieving staff
- be protected, both in terms of responsibility for clients and personally, in the event of accidents.

Why do people volunteer?

It is sometimes of value to discover why individuals wish to be volunteers since it helps to explain their personal motivation and has considerable relevance when considering what they can do. Among the reasons people give for seeking to be volunteer helpers are:

- to be of use to others
- to feel needed
- for social contact and stimulation
- as a way of occupying time
- for personal growth and self-knowledge
- to gain experience prior to seeking paid work as helpers
- to fulfil a personal belief of having something worthwhile to offer
- to offer a specific skill
- because they have relatives in residential care

- because they have been clients themselves
- to fulfil student requirements.

Responsibility for volunteers

A residential facility that plans to embark on a substantial volunteer program will need to designate a member of staff to be responsible for it. The person selected should have sufficient time to ensure the program's success.

Among the responsibilities of a volunteer organiser will be:

> *Recruiting volunteers*
> *Selecting volunteers*
> *Training volunteers*
> *Motivating and supporting volunteers*
> *Resolving difficulties.*

These responsibilities suggest a volunteer organiser should have some seniority in an organisation, broad knowledge of its activities and also personal commitment to the idea of voluntary help.

Recruiting volunteers. Many people who prove to be excellent volunteers do not spontaneously offer their services but do so only when they become aware that a need exists. It follows, therefore, that the supply and availability of volunteers is, for the most part, related to active recruitment programs.

Volunteers can be obtained as a result of a variety of approaches including:

- advertising, for example, through press and television and direct approaches to community organisations
- personal contacts of existing staff and volunteers

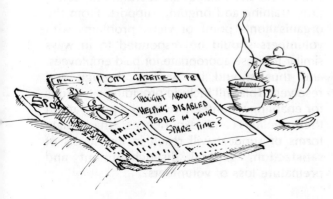

- addressing groups in schools, colleges and community organisations.

Selecting volunteers. Selection should always be based on a formal interview following a visit to a residence by a prospective volunteer. An effective selection process helps to achieve:

- selection of the right kinds of volunteer
- understanding of mutual expectations
- clarification of the time commitment of volunteers and the nature of their contributions to the residence
- understanding of the support volunteers can expect from other workers.

When conducting selection interviews the volunteer organiser may find it helpful to explore the following questions:

- What are the applicant's reasons for wishing to be a volunteer?
- What beliefs does the applicant hold about disabled people?
- Is the applicant appropriately motivated?
- What are the applicant's expectations?
- Is the applicant willing to be directed, trained and supported?
- Is the applicant suited to the tasks he/she may be asked to undertake?
- What skills and personal qualities can the applicant offer?
- Is the applicant likely to be of value to clients?
- How is the applicant likely to get on with staff?
- What can the applicant offer in terms of time commitment?
- Can the applicant act responsibly and retain appropriate confidentiality?

Training volunteers. There should be some basic orientation and initial training program for volunteers as well as ongoing training. It is important to give some input to volunteers prior to deploying them since:

- most are likely to have little knowledge or experience
- what many personally hope to achieve may be inconsistent with the needs of clients

- some may need direction in appropriate behaviour
- some may be inclined to become over-involved or over-committed.

An orientation and initial training program may involve an explanation of:

- general helping approaches to disabled people
- the organisation and its goals
- the needs of clients and how to relate to and help them
- the organisation's expectations of volunteers
- where volunteers will work, and with which staff and clients
- the tasks they will undertake
- ways in which they will be expected to be accountable for what they do and for the time they agree to give
- where they can turn to for help.

Motivating and supporting volunteers. Once volunteers have begun to work in a residence those supporting them should do all they can to ensure that they remain motivated and commited. This can be achieved by:

- giving volunteers something to do which is of value to clients and the organisation
- integrating them into the work situation at an appropriate pace. This may involve working for a time with a member of staff or an experienced volunteer before deciding on their own contribution or accepting responsibility
- ensuring that what they do is personally challenging and rewarding
- ensuring that there is always a person available to help should the need arise
- helping them to see that what they are doing is of benefit to clients
- ensuring that they do not become over-involved as a way of meeting their own needs
- keeping them informed about all relevant aspects of life in the residence
- recognising and developing their contribution

- giving personal feedback on what they are doing
- arranging meetings for sharing experiences and feelings
- ensuring that staff expectations about what volunteers can do are not set too high.

Resolving difficulties. In some organisations the problems volunteers seem to create are considered as being greater than the benefits they have to offer. While this is often more a matter of the attitudes of paid workers than the behaviour of volunteers, difficulties do occasionally occur because some volunteers:

- can be too demanding of employees
- have unenlightened approaches which affect what other helpers are trying to achieve
- are unable to cope with clients
- relate inappropriately to clients
- can, when they are obviously unsuitable, be difficult to ease out of an organisation
- can be unreliable.

There are of course, two sides to the issue of problems. Often, many difficulties are created for volunteers by the organisation. Volunteers can, for example, be:

- taken advantage of
- given inadequate training for tasks assigned to them
- given mundane, unpleasant and unrewarding chores
- given tasks which are too demanding
- given insufficient support and feedback.

Most of these problems are the consequence of an ill-considered approach to volunteers and inadequate recruitment, selection, training and ongoing support. From the organisation's point of view, problems with volunteers should be responded to in ways similar to those appropriate for paid employees, and thus should be worked through and resolved. This will include providing situations for enabling volunteers to speak openly about their feelings and experiences. Inadequate forms of support will result in low levels of satisfaction, general disenchantment and premature loss of volunteers.

14

Special needs

The information contained in this book is of a general nature and is primarily focused upon the adult client. Since, however, residential facilities accommodate children, adolescents and aged people, this chapter briefly explores their more specialised needs.

CHILDREN

At the outset it should be recognised that the needs of disabled children are best met in the context of their own families. This is so because:

- each child requires the affection, security and sense of belonging a family provides
- the family is the most appropriate and effective setting for socialising children
- living in a family is seen as a right and an entitlement.

Wherever possible, forms of help should focus on supporting families so that they are

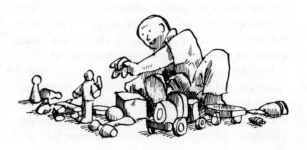

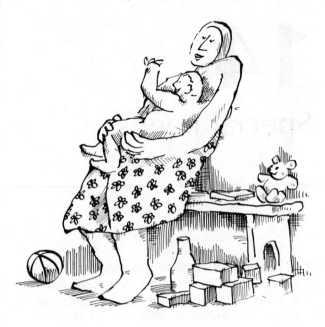

able to care for their disabled children. This may include short-term residential care to:

- meet crisis situations
- give parents relief from the pressures that sometimes accompany the care of a severely disabled child
- undertake assessment and provide forms of help that cannot be carried out at home.

CHILDREN IN RESIDENTIAL SETTINGS

Where parents are unable to care for their children on a longer-term basis, and it is evident that the children are likely to spend their childhood away from their natural families, adoption and fostering should be considered the most acceptable options. Only where exceptional reasons make adoption or fostering impossible should the more usual forms of residential care be considered.

Residential facilities caring for children, however brief or extended the length of stay, should be characterised by an environment and a pattern of relationships which enable essential emotional, developmental and social needs to be met. Each setting should be child centred and will provide:

> *Appropriate parenting*
> *Small group living*
> *A normalised daily life*
> *A context for developing acceptable behaviour*
> *A pattern of life for increasing independence.*

Appropriate parenting

The most important needs of children are met by those adults who care for them. For children living at home these needs will be met by their parents, for those in residential care many should be met by direct care workers. The fact that there are differences between what parents and helpers provide for children may cause some confusion, and so it is of value to clarify the limits of the helping role.

Most children in residential settings have their own parents and so helpers should not seek to take over the provision of those emotional needs associated with the parent–child relationship such as personal identity, attachment and sense of belonging. It is, in fact, unhelpful for helpers to view themselves or to allow others to view them as substitute parents. Not only should children have regular contact with parents, but one of the major responsibilities of the helper is to maintain and enhance relationships between parent and child.

What, then, are the parenting functions that helpers should fulfil? There are two broad areas:

- meeting basic needs for normal healthy development. This includes provision of:
  — food
  — shelter
  — warmth
  — protection
  — personal care
- creating a nurturing climate and intimate caring relationships which enable certain emotional needs to be met, such as the

need for attention, security, recognition and new experiences.

These two areas are interrelated. Meeting basic needs for normal development should take place within a beneficial emotional climate, and a beneficial climate is usually created in the course of meeting basic needs. It will, for example, be at mealtimes, when getting children up, putting them to bed and at bath times where the basis for nurturing relationships will be developed. Daily events such as these are highly significant to children and should generally be characterised by:

- individualised care
- an absence of haste
- open and intimate displays of feeling, tenderness and concern.

Helpers with parenting responsibilities have an obligation to become the kinds of people who are able to meet the emotional and relationship needs of children. They can work towards achieving this by:

- gaining as much knowledge as they can about the physical, emotional and developmental needs of children
- developing ways of functioning so as to be experienced positively on an emotional level. This involves sensitivity to the moods and feelings of children and being able to respond on an immediate basis
- being active in initiating relationships
- seeking comment on their caring styles from those working alongside them.

Meeting the needs of children in organisational contexts is often quite difficult because there are many pressures which seem to undermine a child-centred approach. Perhaps the greatest responsibility helpers have in their parenting role is to safeguard the interests of children by effectively neutralising negative organisational influences. This they can do by:

- viewing their main responsibilities as being to the children in their care and not to employers or colleagues.
- limiting involvement in tasks which intrude

into or undermine the caring role.
- expecting and accepting considerable responsibility for children and their daily program.

Small group living

It is essential for children to be nurtured in the context of small and intimate living groups. Such groups are characterised by:

- geographic separation from adult residences
- a stable group of helpers to make longer-term, secure relationships possible
- the absence of separate facilities for staff such as staff rooms, offices, toilets and bathrooms
- staff wearing ordinary clothes
- staff being known by their names rather than by formal titles
- stimulating conversation and other interactions between children and helpers
- a home-like living environment, that is, one which has the feel of home, is personalised, and has the usual clutter and casualness of home
- a relaxed, stimulating, varied and flexible routine
- a bright and cheerful environment, created and changed by staff and children
- plenty of toys and games which are always accessible to children
- access for children to kitchens and to drinks and snacks
- an open invitation for children to bring friends home.

Normalised daily life

In addition to the points discussed in the previous section, a normalised daily life will involve:

- a daily routine that is like that of other children in society
- normal daily activities such as attending kindergarten or going to school
- the involvement of children in everyday

domestic routines such as shopping, preparation of meals and household chores
- regular outings
- special occasions
- opportunities for children to play with staff,
  with each other, with their friends and by
  themselves.

Developing acceptable behaviour

Socialising children involves the creation of
boundaries for the development of appropriate behaviour. Residential situations should
aim to provide environments that establish
these boundaries but which are, at the same
time, sufficiently flexible to permit and
encourage individuality and self-determination. In family situations, a satisfactory
balance between imposed boundaries, on the
one hand, and self-determination, on the
other, is rarely achieved. Against a background of the needs of the developing child,
stability is probably unattainable. Where
parents and children have been able to establish some kind of understanding and a
mutually satisfying balance, it has usually been
a consequence of commitment and effort over
a long period of time. In most residential
contexts, because of the duration of care and
the changing situation as far as staff is
concerned, it is rarely possible to achieve an
entirely satisfying balance. It is important for
staff to realise this and to accept that a certain
degree of conflict is inherent in the socialisation of children.

One of the realities of much residential care
of children is that many employed in caring
roles have little previous experience and few
skills. Motivated by a belief that they personally have a great deal to offer, they tend,
without realising it, to set quite unrealistic
standards and to demand an unreasonable
degree of compliance. When children do not
respond in the desired ways, helpers often
experience a sense of failure and disillusionment. Sometimes this can make them quite
hostile to children.

It is essential for helpers to appreciate that
many of the difficulties they encounter in
caring for children are a consequence, not of
something inherent in the children, but of
their own expectations and lack of appreciation of the needs of the growing child. No
children, including those who are disabled,
have inbuilt devices to tell them to obey
adults and be compliant. What they want for
themselves and what carers want for them is
frequently quite different, and the expression
of disagreement and challenge should be seen
as normal. When it occurs, discussion and
negotiation should be the usual responses.
Thus, the task of socialising children is not
one of moulding them according to some
predetermined and arbitrary set of ideas but
of creating a pattern of life based on tolerance, the expression of feeings and the resolution of disagreements.

Increasing independence

Care of disabled children has in the past been
characterised by total dependence on helpers.
Contemporary approaches are built on the
belief that they should have all necessary
opportunities to develop to the limits of their

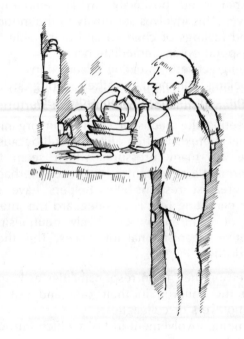

ability. Within residential facilities this will entail:

- enabling them to have a wider range of choice
- allowing them greater freedom and risk
- giving and expecting greater responsibility
- tolerating, accepting and accommodating their opinions
- accommodating their differences in behaviour and living standards.

At the same time, practices for increasing the independence of disabled children should not differ from those which are typical for children living in their own homes. While it is impossible to generalise about standards of child care, the behaviour of many parents suggest that they do not expect their children to become independent too quickly but seek to provide them with a certain degree of indulgence. Even though most children of eight, for example, are capable of bathing themselves, parents may be involved because of the pleasure it gives and the meaning it has for both them and their children.

In mainstream society one of the pleasures of being a child is that there is always someone nearby who is warm, caring and interested, who will help you get up in the morning, dress you, provide you with meals, make a fuss of you, create a sense of fun, take your side, be there when you are unhappy and tolerate your swings in mood. Probably thousands of children have been raised in residential situations without such nurturing and have suffered as a consequence. Since this kind of attention appears to be integral to notions of good child care in western society, it should not be denied to disabled children who live away from home.

Many of the personal needs of children should, then, be met by staff, even where children have the potential to take care of themselves. This means that helpers, while actively caring for and nurturing them, will, at the same time, unobtrusively ensure that they acquire the necessary developmental skills and degrees of independence.

ADOLESCENTS

Adolescence is a stage of transition from the dependence of the child to the independence of the adult. In western societies it is seen as a difficult stage not only for young people themselves but also for their families and the wider society because:

- it is a stage of heightened personal awareness
- it is a time for developing an identity which involves an acute concern for:
  — appearance
  — personal and sexual attractiveness
  — appropriateness
  — peer acceptance.
- it is a stage of considerable experimentation
- it is a time of idealism, certainty and often impatience
- it is a time when personal values are often at variance with those of adults.

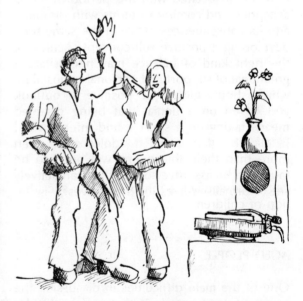

Disabled adolescents living in residential accommodation should be able to enjoy a pattern of life that is no different from that of their able counterparts in the community. This means that helpers will assist in ways that take account of the realities and stresses that characterise this period of life.

Enabling adolescents to become increasingly independent will involve:

- providing them with appropriate opportunities for making decisions and choices
- giving them greater power and control of their lives
- enabling them to have greater freedom within and beyond a residence
- responding in open and non-judgemental ways when discussing personal standards and beliefs
- ensuring that they have greater privacy
- allowing freedom to develop interests that are normal for adolescents
- letting them experiment with ideas, behaviour, forms of dress, etc. that are part of adolescent culture
- tolerating and understanding changes in mood.

For the disabled adolescent, an additional difficulty associated with this period of life is accepting and coming to terms with disability and its consequences, while at the same time developing a positive self-concept. Achieving the right kind of balance may necessitate a great deal of support and personal counselling which should always be positive in outlook and based on a denial that being disabled means taking on a specific and inferior role. It may be that disabled adolescents, even more than their able peers, will need to be taught to be assertive so that they can actively seek normalised lives for themselves.

AGED PEOPLE

One of the main difficulties in discussing the needs of aged people is that social attitudes usually place all those beyond their mid-sixties in this category. The reason for so doing is closely related both to the value, or rather lack of value, accorded to individuals when they pass normal retirement age and to incorrect assumptions about their needs. Society appears to hold the view that aged people:

- usually suffer from ill health
- wish to have a life which is restful and where no demands are made of them
- do not want to live with younger people
- should live in a 'home'
- are incapable of doing much that is meaningful.

When considering the needs of older people, be it in the wider society or in the context of residential care, it is unhelpful to think in terms of one group. Between the ages of sixty-five and eighty-five are people with widely differing needs and capabilities; what someone, for example, in their late sixties desires and is capable of achieving may be quite different from someone twenty years older, although even here there are dangers in generalisation.

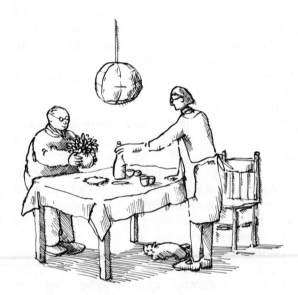

Older people, no less than others, and quite irrespective of age, need a life where they are active and fully involved in the world around them. Being advanced in years and also disabled should not lead to assumptions about incapability or a need for total care. Most disabled elderly people living in residential accommodation are capable of doing a great deal for themselves, and so their pattern of daily life should not be that of the hotel where everything is done for them, nor should it be like a hospital where they are treated as sick. In principle, it should be no different from that of younger age groups, so involving them in:

- planning, organising and making decisions about their lives, particularly what they do on a day-to-day basis
- daily tasks such as preparation of food, setting tables, gardening, washing, domestic chores and shopping. These are the kinds of activities older people living in their own homes are involved in and which, without

realising it, often give a sense of purpose and meaningfully occupy time.

Older clients, like others, should live in small groups, and the aim will be to continue to care for them within such groups as they become more infirm. Both the tradition of accommodating them in hospital-like settings, and the newer practice of moving them from situation to situation as they become more infirm has a certain administrative convenience, and seems rational where they are understood only in terms of health needs, but the major consequence is to destroy most other areas of their lives which are of significance to them.

15

Education, work and leisure needs

Education, work and leisure needs of disabled people are quite distinct topics and are grouped together in this chapter only for convenience. Had consideration of them been more comprehensive they would have merited separate chapters.

The three areas do, however, have a great deal in common:

- they are significant aspects of life
- each occupies large parts of the day and has the potential to give it meaning
- they are essential aspects of a more normalised life
- they are areas from which most disabled people have, in the past, been excluded
- they are aspects of life to which disabled people have an entitlement
- in each area there is a need to achieve positive discrimination in favour of disabled people and to take action if they are discriminated against
- they are areas where the concept of least restrictive alternative has relevance.

Meeting work, education and leisure needs of disabled people is, for the most part, beyond the direct control of helpers in residential facilities. There is much, however, that helpers can do to foster client involvement and success in these important areas of life, and this chapter seeks to make some appropriate suggestions.

EDUCATION

Children with disabilities have traditionally been excluded from mainstream education, because they have been considered either incapable of learning or as having needs that can only be met in specialised facilities. As a result, a range of educational and residential facilities have been developed expressly to meet their perceived needs. Despite what they have offered, these facilities are now seen as having had quite negative consequences for many children. Not only have they sustained abnormal conceptions of them, they have denied disabled children opportunities to develop appropriately through mixing with non-disabled children in normal schools.

Today, the emphasis is on integrating children into normal schools, and this trend is described as mainstreaming. The philosophy of mainstreaming does not, however, assert that all disabled children should attend normal schools — some may always need special day or residential forms of education — but that many at present in special schools would be better helped in schools in the community if the necessary resources and forms of support were made available.

In residences caring for children of school age, helpers may need to take on advocate roles concerning the issue of access to mainstream education. Where it is evident that disabled children are capable of being integrated, but little is being done to achieve it, helpers should consider exerting pressure on education authorities and also, where necessary, on particular schools.

Supporting children at school

In whatever schools children are placed, helpers should get to know and work closely with teachers to ensure that children receive all the help they need and are dealt with appropriately. This can be achieved by:

- establishing contact with the head teacher
- meeting regularly with teachers to explore any difficulties children may be encountering and to discuss progress
- taking up with teachers treatment of disabled children which appears to be discriminatory
- becoming familiar with the subjects children are studying
- providing additional educational help in the living environment for those needing it
- encouraging school personnel to contact helpers where difficulties arise.

The pattern of life of a residence should seek to support what happens at school. This is likely to involve:

- providing a lifestyle that encourages learning
- generally supporting schools and teachers in discussions which children
- ensuring that children have all they require to succeed at school, including uniforms, necessary books, stationery, equipment and finance for trips and holidays
- ensuring that children can attend all school activities
- helping children with homework.

School life, both in terms of learning and social experiences, is a major part of an individual's socialisation process and is highly significant in contributing to the quality of adult life. Children who succeed at school

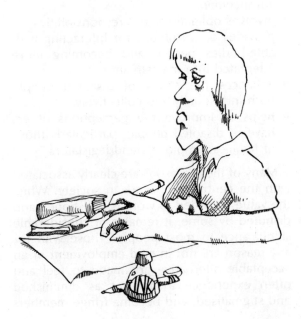

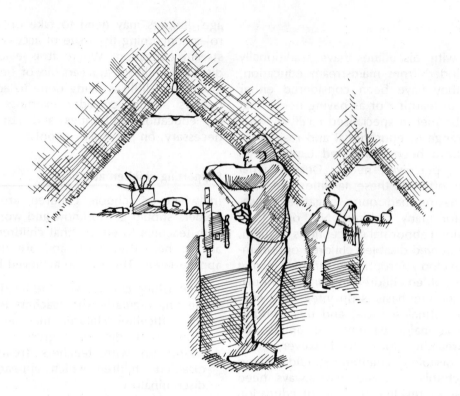

usually have concerned adults behind them who are not only supportive but who work with and occasionally pressurise schools to ensure that educational experiences are of value. Disabled children need this kind of support as much as, if not more than, other groups of disadvantaged children.

WORK

This section explores the place of work in the lives of disabled people together with a number of related issues. Since many clients in residential accommodation attend some kind of day centre, meeting their employment or occupation needs will involve close co-operation between residence and day centre.

As is the case with other members of society, disabled adults have a basic right to paid employment because it:

- is a normal feature of life
- is used as a measure for evaluating the worth of an individual

- provides an earned income, the disposal of which is the individual's responsibility
- provides meaning and purpose, and offers opportunities for attaining personal satisfaction and a sense of achievement and advancement
- involves obligations and responsibilities
- provides opportunities for interacting with able-bodies people and becoming more integrated into mainstream society
- enhances the status of disabled people both individually and collectively
- helps to improve the perceptions others have of disabled people, particularly those of families, employers and legislators.

Many of these reasons are clearly associated with the centrality of work in society. While the value accorded to work is questioned and disputed by some, it remains of considerable significance to most people. Those who for any reason are not in paid employment or an acceptable alternative are made to feel and often experience themselves as diminished and stigmatised, and become fringe members of society. Since present approaches to disabled people reflect mainstream social beliefs, appropriate efforts should be made to integrate disabled people into the workforce.

Work in congregate facilities

The majority of disabled people living in congregate residences, apart from those with the most profound disabilities, have always worked. For the most part, however, the work they have undertaken has been related to the maintenance of residential facilities, thus they have been used in kitchens and laundries, to remove refuse and on farms and gardens. Much of this work has been of a menial kind and offered few possibilities for attaining any real job satisfaction or recognition. Perhaps, more importantly, it was almost always unpaid.

The exploitation of clients by compelling them to work without pay is known as peonage. The original meaning of this term related to the practice of holding debtors in servitude to work off debts and convicts to make amends for their crimes. Although past forms of treatment of disabled people were never devised with such intentions, the consequences of indefinite detention in institutions and imposed work gave clients a status that was little different from that of debtor or convict.

The practice of using clients as unpaid labour to operate residences is something that should be abandoned. Where clients choose to work in this way, and it is consistent with their individual plans and does not exploit them, payment should always be made.

Reality of work for disabled people

As was stated at the beginning of this section, disabled people have as much right to paid work as do others, and both society in general and helpers involved in assisting them have a responsibility to do all they can to make it possible. The reality is, however, that although the exclusion of disabled people from the work force has been related more to social attitudes than to capabilities, both the present competitive nature of open employment and decline in available jobs make it probable that many are unlikely ever to find work. This does not mean that helpers should resign themselves to the exclusion of clients from the work force, but that they should balance efforts to prepare them for work and to find jobs against the possibility that they will be unsuccessful. Thus, while pursuing open employment, encouraging self-employment or other work-related enterprises, helpers should, at the same time, be exploring with clients rewarding alternative lifestyles.

Work in open employment

There is overwhelming evidence to indicate that most disabled people have the capacity to perform quite complex work tasks, and that they are no less reliable than able-bodied people. The issue of whether they have the potential to work should not, then, be in question. But because of resistance to their employment it has always been difficult for them to obtain work, and many, having been unemployed for most of their adult lives, have never developed adequate skills for entry into and survival in the workforce.

If clients are to be successfully employed there are a number of ways they should be assisted by helpers. Among them are:

> *Clarifying feelings and hopes about work*
> *Obtaining information about jobs*
> *Preparation for entry into the workforce*
> *Preparation for specific jobs*
> *Support at work.*

Clarifying feelings and hopes about work

Clients with no previous substantial work experience can become more aware of the realities of work through discussions, visits to work situations and by observing the kinds of jobs to which they feel attracted. Success at this stage will be dependent upon the knowledge helpers have of the kinds of problems disabled people tend to encounter at work

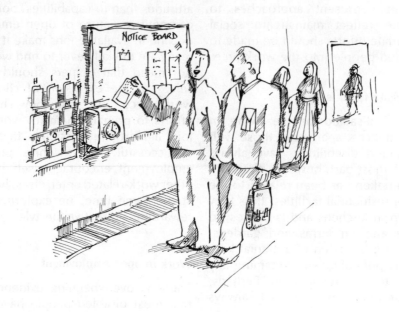

and of the occupations suited to them. In relation to the latter point, the range of occupations in which physically disabled people have successfully been employed is as varied as that for able-bodied members of society. For those with intellectual disabilities, the range is also wide. Among the jobs they have succeeded in have been:

- *gardening*
- *farm labouring*
- *kitchen work*
- *upholstery*
- *assembling*
- *picture framing*
- *painting and decorating*
- *office cleaning*
- *car washing*
- *packing*
- *printing*
- *portering*
- *cement and brick work.*

Obtaining information about jobs

This involves establishing links with government departments and local businesses to promote the employment of disabled people and to learn of job opportunities as they arise.

It may also involve working to modify beliefs employers have about the kinds of jobs disabled people are able to do, and discussions on the forms of support that can be provided to enable disabled people to be successfully employed.

Efforts such as these may occasionally result in the offer of work on condition that clients are appropriately prepared and trained. It is therefore necessary to identify the skills a

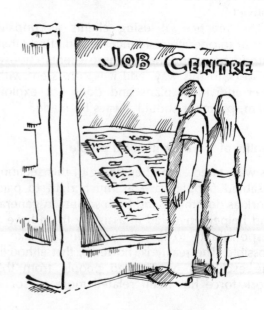

specific job entails and this is likely to involve observation of those people presently undertaking it.

Preparation for entry into the workforce

The task of training people for entry into the workforce will, as has been indicated, be preceded by an assessment of their capabilities together with the range of supports, both direct and indirect, that may be required to enable them to work successfully in particular settings.

A specific pre-work training program may involve developing client skills in areas such as:

- job application and interview skills
- timekeeping and punctuality
- mobility, and perhaps use of public transport
- personal presentation
- ability to follow instructions
- ability to complete tasks
- appropriate role behaviour
- general literacy skills.

Preparation for specific jobs

The extent to which preparation is necessary will vary according to the needs of clients and work settings. Among the areas that may be worth considering are:

- an employment agreement, including the possibility of a trial period
- introduction to work on a part-time basis
- provision of aids and personal assistance to clients at work

Support at work

Staff should give a great deal of support to clients when they enter open employment for the first time. This may, for example, involve transporting them for the first few weeks even where they have the ability to get to work unaided. Support should also be available to an employer, initially through regular contact and discussion.

Sheltered work

Various forms of day services, such as adult training centres, activity therapy centres and sheltered workshops, exist to offer both occupation and other experiences to disabled people. Where it is appropriate for them to do so, these facilities should be used to prepare clients for open employment or, alternatively, they can provide opportunities for gainful employment in more protected settings.

Unemployment

Some disabled people will be incapable of working or may, because of immense personal and social barriers, not wish to. Rather than continually create a feeling that they ought to work, it would be more beneficial to accept their exclusion from the workforce. For such clients alternatives should be developed which have the potential to offer considerable personal rewards, and this is an issue that is considered in the next section.

LEISURE

Leisure can be understood in terms of what people do with their free time. For most, that time is limited as a result of other demands and commitments, particularly those associated with employment. While many people see their leisure activities as of considerable importance, leisure usually has meaning only in relation to those other demands. Were they to have greater time available, it would not necessarily follow that it would be given to leisure pursuits. Indeed, it may bring about a loss of interest. The weekend artist, for example, may not be interested in painting full-time and may, when much more time becomes available, give up the activity entirely.

Leisure and unemployment

There is a need to be clear about the nature of leisure because it is often assumed to have

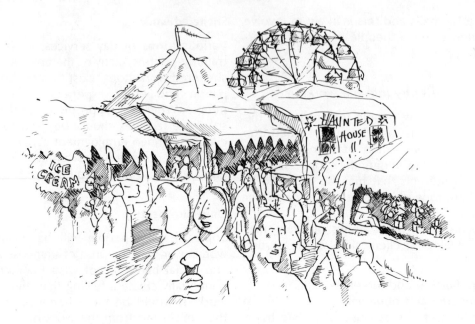

greater significance for disabled people than for others. The preceding discussion on work has suggested that many disabled people face the possibility of being permanently excluded from the work force. This has consequences for the total pattern of their lives, the way they live on a day-to-day basis and the use of time. If many are to be denied the chance of regular work, it is important that the psychological and time gaps unemployment creates are compensated for by some purposeful activity. Because of the essential nature of leisure, it would be false to believe that most disabled people can become satisfied and achieve a sense of fulfilment merely by spending greater time in leisure pursuits. Helpers may need to assist clients in developing interests in quite new areas where there is a potential to provide meaning on a long-term basis, and this may include responsible roles in residential settings and voluntary work.

Importance of leisure

Leisure pursuits are higly valued in western societies. They are considered to be central to the well-being and self-fulfilment of individuals, and an essential dimension in the development of the total person. Leisure essentially means doing those things one chooses and wants to do, in time not given to other areas of life, because they may be of interest, be pleasurable, offer stimulation, be a form of discovery and exploration, or a way of helping and giving to others. Table 15.1 indicates some of the leisure pursuits enjoyed by disabled people.

Table 15.1 Leisure pursuits

Cricket	Athletics
Swimming	Handball
Netball	Skittles
Tennis	Ten pin bowling
Volleyball	Bowls
Roller skating	Billards and snooker
Darts	Record libraries
Gymnastics	Toys and table games
Putting	Cinema
Weightlifting	Dominoes
Camping	Mime and drama
Canoeing	Puppetry
Keep fit	Art
Trampoline	Music
Table tennis	Theatre
Card games	Computers
Dancing	Scouts and Rangers
Riding	Rambler clubs
Archery	Parties
Guides	Internal radio
Women's institutes	Keeping pets and other animals
Youth clubs	such as fish, chickens,
Football	hamsters, mice, donkeys,
Badminton	goats, guinea-pigs, birds,
Reading	tortoises

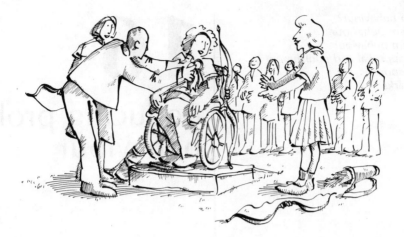

Normalising leisure

Leisure and recreation activities for disabled people should, wherever possible, be normalised, that is, they should be provided in ways that are no different from mainstream society. This means that disabled people should:

- be involved in leisure pursuits that are age-appropriate
- be able to pursue activities where a normal degree of risk is involved
- not be discriminated against by community groups but have equal access to community-based leisure activities
- be helped to acquire leisure and social skills that will enhance integration
- not have leisure activities organised in a way that isolates them from mainstream society

- not have leisure pursuits defined as therapy
- wherever appropriate, participate with staff in leisure activities.

For helpers in residential settings this means that they will need to:

- ensure that clients participate in some leisure activities on an individual basis rather than in the company of a number of disabled people
- ensure that adequate transport is available, or that clients have the skills for independent travel
- offer appropriate and necessary support and assistance to community groups where disabled people are involved.

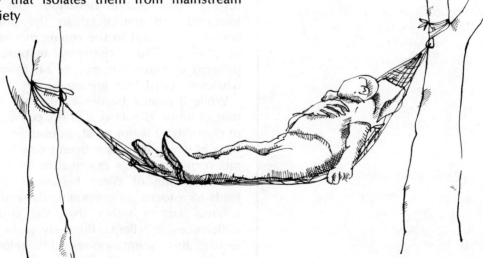

16

Reducing problem behaviour

This chapter discusses a range of issues associated with client behaviour that helpers view as problematic or unacceptable. Underlying discussion is an assumption that if clients live in normalised environments and enjoy supportive and helpful relationships, their behaviour will not differ markedly from that of others. Since many clients, however, have never experienced such environments or relationships they will have developed quite inappropriate ways of behaving. A belief still shared by many workers in congregated residences is that extreme client behaviour is an inevitable consequence of disability, thus it is to be viewed, not as something which can be changed, but as the realities around which residential life should be structured. As a result, unacceptable behaviour has been tolerated and reinforced to the point of becoming integral to the coping mechanisms of clients. Thus, changing inappropriate patterns of behaviour may be far from easy, whatever approaches are used.

While it cannot be denied that the behaviour of some clients is a direct consequence of disability, it is, for most, an outcome of the ways in which they have been treated. Recognition of this fact is essential to an accurate understanding of client behaviour since it leads to a focus on environmental and interactional factors rather than the supposed deficiences in clients themselves. In other words, this orientation enables helpers to respond to causes rather than to symtoms and to search for ways of adapting the environment and pattern of life to the benefit of clients.

Whatever the nature of client behaviour, before helpers consider taking action they should:

> *Ensure they are operating from appropriate definitions of what is and is not problem behaviour*
> *Attempt to identify specific factors causing problem behaviour.*

WHAT IS PROBLEM BEHAVIOUR?

What constitutes appropriate and inappropriate behaviour in the residential context may seem so self-evident that an examination of it seems superfluous. A list such as that in the right hand column of Table 16.1 appears to indicate quite clearly what it is. While there is much to support this argument, identifying problem behaviour is, in fact, often not a simple but a quite complex process because:

- most problem behaviour is an outcome of transactions between clients and others, and not deficiencies in clients themselves. This means that those transactions should be open to scrutiny
- definitions of unacceptable behaviour are usually based on the personal standards and values of helpers and these, too, should be open to scrutiny
- the right of helpers to control the behaviour of adult disabled people is in itself questionable.

It must be the case, therefore, that when attempting to establish standards in residential contexts, some basic principles should be followed. For example, standards should:

- result from discussion involving staff and clients
- reflect the developmental needs of clients and be age-appropriate
- be consistent with what is generally considered as normal for intimate living situations

Table 16.1 Environmental factors and problem behaviour

Environmental factors	Consequent behaviour
Containment and isolation of clients, e.g. fences, locked doors, rigid rules and routine	absconding, frustration and boredom, emotional withdrawal, questionable sexual behaviour
Denial of privacy, e.g. large dormitories, no curtains, no locks, constant surveillance	public displays of inappropriate behaviour, unacceptable attempts to create privacy by excluding staff
Lack of stimulation and purposeful activity, e.g. drab environment, long periods of inactivity, meaningless client relationships	destructive acts, self-mutilation, self-stimulation, e.g. flicking hands, continual masturbation, obsessive behaviour
Denial of age-appropriate behaviour, e.g. infantilism, no personal responsibility or choice	disobedience, obstructiveness, violence, regressive behaviour
Staff dominance, e.g. directive, punitive, brutal, disinterested	general hostility and resistance, obsequiousness, avoidable incontinence, inability to make decisions for self, no standards in hygiene or self-care, no spontaneity, stereotyped behaviour
Denial of personal identity, e.g. institutional clothes, no possessions	theft and destruction of property
Punitive treatment, e.g. isolation, detention, enforced medication, deprivation, abuse	retaliatory violence, escapist behaviour, violence to other clients

- never be permanent but open to discussion and negotiation whenever clients and helpers wish to question or challenge them
- never be attained through compulsion or abnormal degrees of psychological manipulation.

CAUSES OF PROBLEM BEHAVIOUR

This section explores a number of ways of explaining the origins of problem behaviour. While each is considered separately for ease of understanding, much problem behaviour will, in reality, be caused or be sustained by a combination of these factors and so they should not be seen as mutually exclusive. The possible causes of problem behaviour considered are:

> *Personal disability*
> *Helper expectations*
> *Learned helplessness*
> *The nature of institutional life.*

Personal disability

Much of the behaviour of some disabled people that would be viewed as problematic or abnormal in others is a consequence of their disabilities, for example:

- clumsiness
- frustrations arising from physical restrictions
- conflict in relationships as a result of an inability to accurately perceive what is going on.

Helper expectations

Standards used by helpers to establish patterns of daily life and to define appropriate and inappropriate behaviour vary greatly from residence to residence. When these standards are inappropriate or unrealistic they can in themselves be a major cause of problem behaviour. Among such standards are those which:

- are too high. Where staff operate with standards that are unattainable or expect clients to behave in ways that are contrary to their personal and interpersonal needs, difficulties are bound to arise
- are too low. Many approaches to disabled people, as has already been indicated, are based on beliefs suggesting an inability to be other than primitive and anti-social. In consequence, standards set by helpers have been so low as to virtually encourage clients to develop abnormally
- expect total conformity. In some settings helpers have demanded total conformity

from clients and have reacted punitively when it has not been forthcoming. In addition to the fact that, as has been suggested, unattainable standards inevitably lead to conflict, the natural desire of clients to control their lives cannot but create confrontations with helpers
- deny the reality of shared living. Situations where people live together are characterised by frequent difficulties and disagreements, and occasional periods of stress. Helpers in residential facilities often fail to recognise that these dimensions are part of normal daily life and as natural for disabled people living together as they are for others. Sometimes this denial is a consequence of the public nature of residential life, and an expectation on the part of senior staff that direct care workers should run trouble-free residences. Whatever the reason, the efforts of staff to provide clients with tranquil lives by eliminating all conflict are not only unreasonable, but they can be experienced by clients as oppressive.

Learned helplessness

There is considerable evidence to indicate that inconsistency in treatment over a period of time renders people helpless. Where children, for example, live in unstable and unpredictable environments, are treated by adults in conflicting ways, such as being rewarded and punished at different times for identical behaviour, they will fail to learn the relationship between cause and effect or between behaviour and its consequences. They will therefore be unable to respond appropriately however they are dealt with and so, in effect, will become helpless.

Such a lack of consistency is common in many residential settings and its consequence for clients has been to render them helpless. This is often the reason why the most severe forms of punishment fail to have any effect.

Institutional life

Perhaps the most useful way of drawing some

of these explanations together and making sense of them is to understand problem behaviour in relation to the task assigned to the institution. Since about the beginning of this century, if not before that time, institutions were seen as warehouses for containing many of society's undesirable people. As a result, it was not surprising that they developed negative and depriving regimes which, as far as disabled people were concerned, produced adjustment behaviour far in excess of that which was a natural outcome of disability (see Table 16.1). The role of custodian assigned to staff and the definitions of disabled people prevailing at the time, prevented an understanding of the real causes of client behaviour. Within a relatively short space of time the belief that extreme behaviour was a consequence of disability became indelibly fixed in the minds of all who worked in institutions. Each new generation of staff was immediately confronted by such behaviour and, not having the capacity to question conventional wisdom, naturally assumed it to be an outcome of disability. Thus the contain-

ment goal of the institution, together with the lack of understanding on the part of staff, produced a pattern of life characterised by outrageous client behaviour and punitive and repressive staff responses. Once a pattern of this kind had been established, both inmates and custodians were trapped by it. Such a situation is suggested in Figure 16.1.

REDUCING PROBLEM BEHAVIOUR

When problem behaviour has reached the point where helpers consider it essential to take some action they should:

> *Ensure they have an accurate understanding of the behaviour in question Respond appropriately and effectively.*

Clarifying unacceptable behaviour

Surprising though it may seem, helpers often have a superficial understanding of the behaviour they consider unacceptable. Sometimes

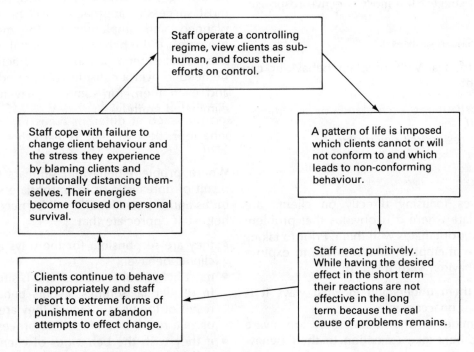

Fig. 16.1 Institution-centred environment and problem behaviour.

they hear about it in rather dramatic conversations with colleagues, do not challenge what is said and build up quite distorted images. Attempts to deal with problem behaviour must be based on a realistic understanding and appraisal of it, and this will include asking such questions as:

- Exactly what behaviour is unacceptable?
- Why is it thought to be unacceptable?
- Who is asserting it to be unacceptable?
- How often does it occur?
- What precedes its occurrence?
- What are its consequences?
- How do others respond?
- In what way do the responses of others reinforce it?
- What appears to be the cause?
- What is the significance of the behaviour for the client?

It may be helpful to keep a record of the behaviour and to identify exact reasons for considering it to be unacceptable. Not only will this lead to a more accurate picture of what is happening to a client or group of clients, it is likely to result in a level of analysis that will suggest the most effective response.

Appropriate responses

Action to deal with problem behaviour can focus on:

> Clients
> Staff
> The residential environment.

Clients

Responses focusing directly on clients are appropriate where it is obvious that problem behaviour originates with them. Prior to taking action an attempt should be made to explore their behaviour with them to:

- help them understand in what ways it is seen as unacceptable
- determine to what extent they are aware that others take exception to their behaviour

- indicate what their behaviour does to others
- identify what they feel to be the cause of their behaviour
- find out whether they wish to change, and if they do the assistance they would find helpful
- work out a program of help.

For clients with little insight or understanding helpers can, by becoming aware of the occasions and situations when problem behaviour tends to occur:

- reduce or eliminate the circumstances giving rise to it
- keep its impact to a minimum when it does occur
- ensure that the way in which they respond does not reinforce it.

Whether or not clients have any awareness of the effects of their actions on others, responses should concentrate on teaching appropriate behaviour rather than on eliminating inappropriate behaviour, that is, rewarding that which is desired rather than punishing that which is inappropriate. The most successful approaches will be carefully planned and implemented by means of programs. If the behaviour is central to clients and sustains their self-identities, action may be needed over a considerable period of time and even then, for some, it may never be eliminated entirely.

Staff

Where problem behaviour appears to be a result of unrealistic or inappropriate staff attitudes and expectations, it will be necessary to help staff appreciate that:

- they are responsible for the ways in which clients behave
- most behaviour is learned and is situational. In residential settings, clients behave as a result of the ways in which they are treated or as a result of a modelling process
- if they wish the behaviour of clients to be different, they may first need to change

their own behaviour

- they should be able to tolerate and accept behaviour in clients that differs from their own personal standards
- bargaining and negotiation are essential aspects of residential life.

In addition to enabling helpers to have greater appreciation of the many factors contributing to problem behaviour, they should be assisted in developing skills to identify client need and to respond in helpful ways. This is likely to involve:

- their attendance at client planning meetings
- teaching them how to build closer relationships with clients, to achieve greater reciprocity and to become more appropriate models
- encouraging them to present for discussion

at staff meetings any difficulties they experience in understanding or relating to clients

- providing supportive contexts to enable them to discuss each other's caring style
- helping them to acquire skills so as to avoid unnecessary confrontations and difficult episodes, and to deal with them effectively when they occur.

Residential environment

The general contents of this book and particularly ideas in Chapter 10 describe the characteristics of residential environments that are client centred. When such environments exist they have a marked impact on client behaviour as Figure 16.2 attempts to convey.

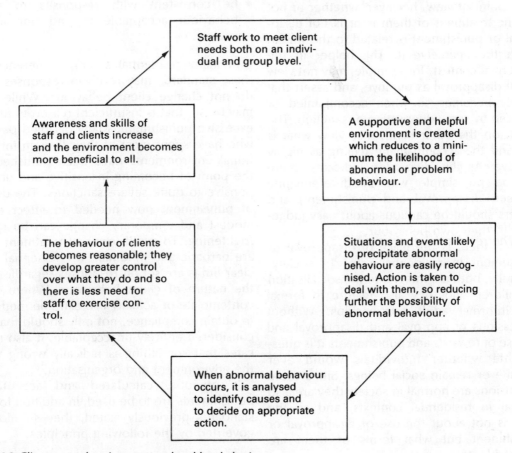

Fig. 16.2 Client-centred environment and problem behaviour.

THE PLACE OF DISAPPROVAL AND PUNISHMENT

Problem behaviour in residential situations will be eliminated or reduced to normal dimensions where, as has been argued, both the quality of the living environment and staff–client interactions reflect client need. In seeking to create a beneficial pattern of life the question arises as to the place of disapproval and punishment. Does disapproval and punishment have any part to play in residential life?

Before attempting to answer this question it is necessary to explore what is meant by disapproval and punishment. From an objective point of view these concepts can be explored in terms of a continuum, from the mildest forms of disapproval to the most severe forms of punishment. From the recipients' point of view, however, whether or not specific treatment of them is or is not disapproval or punishment is related to the way in which they perceive it. The helper in the residential context, for example, may not view verbal disapproval as punitive, and assert that it only becomes so when accompanied or replaced by some deprivation or sanction. The client, on the other hand, may view what is said and the accompanying feeling as highly punitive. As this discussion indicates, there can be no simple way of differentiating between disapproval and punishment, and helpers should be cautious about easy judgement of their own behaviour.

What, then, is the place of disapproval or punishment in residential care? In society, generally, both are integral to the socialisation of children and they also feature in formal and informal adult relationships. Without expressions of approval and disapproval and the use of rewards and punishments it is questionable whether individuals would ever become or remain social beings. Since these dimensions are normal in society they are also normal in residential contexts, and so the issue is not about the use of disapproval or punishment but what forms of them are acceptable.

While it is impossible to propose general rules, negative responses to disabled people should:

- be appropriate to the age, sex and level of functioning of clients
- be appropriate to the context in which they are being used, that is, residence, school, work or social situation
- reflect a respect for the integrity and dignity of the clients involved
- enable clients to understand why they are being treated in a particular way and to learn greater discrimination between acceptable and unacceptable behaviour
- be in the context of ongoing helping relationships
- be effective
- not exceed the response the behaviour merits
- be consistent with responses to such behaviour acceptable to and normal in society.

In many residential settings adherence to these standards may result in responses that do not change client behaviour. While this may be so, that is insufficient reason to justify excessive punishment. Many disabled people who have spent most of their lives in institutional environments have been punished to the point of becoming insensitive and unresponsive to quite severe sanctions. The degree of punishment now needed to effect even modest and temporary change can be quite frightening. To avoid forms of treatment that are barbaric and inhuman, it is essential that clear limits are set on responses regardless of the nature of client behaviour. Where staff contemplate or actually use extreme methods to obtain compliance, not only should that be considered entirely unacceptable, it also indicates that something is radically wrong with the environment and organisation.

If obvious, calculated and acceptable punishments are to be used, in addition to the standards previously stated, they should be governed by the following principles:

- the behaviour the punishment seeks to

correct should be clearly defined and stated
- the punishment should be used as close in time as possible to the behaviour
- it should be used consistently and without exception
- it should not be administered by a worker in an angry or frustrated state
- it should not humiliate, frighten or belittle a client nor effect emotional or physical harm
- the worker administering it should have a significant relationship with the client and be able, on other occasions, to reward appropriate behaviour

UNACCEPTABLE RESPONSES

Certain responses to client behaviour should today be viewed as unacceptable because they:

- are morally or ethically untenable
- inflict harm on clients by:
  - evoking extreme levels of anxiety and fear
  - eliciting avoidance behaviour that can be more disturbing and problematic than the behaviour warranting punishment
  - negatively affecting a client's self-concept
  - producing hostility and aggression towards those effecting the punishment
- are inconsistent with contemporary values about the worth of human beings
- are usually unsuccessful in bringing about permanent change in client behaviour.
  Among such unacceptable responses are:

  Inappropriate use of medication
  Physical restraint
  Isolation
  Denial of regular meals
  Verbal abuse
  Client control
  Corporal punishment.

Inappropriate use of medication

The use of medication to control behaviour

may sometimes by necessary. There are many conditions that can lead to disturbed behaviour if not treated, and so medication is clearly a valid form of treatment. At the same time, its use should always be challenged when prescribed following problem behaviour, because that behaviour may have external causes.

While the responsibility for prescribing any form of medication rests with a medical practitioner, if it is desired to suppress certain behaviour, it should not be prescribed until discussions involving the client, appropriate relatives and helpers have taken place and there is agreement that it would be of benefit. These discussions will also consider any side-effects of medication to be used. Once medication has been prescribed, its use should be reviewed within six weeks and then at regular intervals afterwards.

Physical restraint

In situations of extreme violence, immediate short-term restraint may be necessary to protect clients from themselves or others from them. There will be few occasions, however, where its use should be sustained for any period time.

When physical restraint is resorted to:

- the degree of force used should be the minimum necessary to attain control
- it should be used in a way that seeks to calm rather than provoke
- there should be sufficient staff available to avoid injury to any person involved
- it should be effected wherever possible by holding clothing
- a record should be made of the incident and the kind of restraint used
- a meeting following the incident should be held to analyse the circumstances leading to its use, and to find ways of avoiding recurrence.

Isolation

Isolation, like physical restraint, may occasionally be necessary. When it is used:

- it should be for the shortest period of time possible
- it should be in a reasonable environment
- the client should not be left unattended
- a record should be made of circumstances leading to its use, the behaviour of the client when isolated and the period of time involved.

Denial of meals

The denial of meals should never be considered an acceptable form of punishment, and even the practice of delaying meals to achieve desired behaviour should be questioned if it is resorted to frequently.

Verbal abuse

While banter and humourous insults may be part of many ongoing relationships, practices such as abusive shouting, ridicule, insults, swearing, the dictatorial issuing of orders or intimidation should not be seen as acceptable forms of response. Staff should discipline themselves in the use of offensive language to gain control, even when they justify it as being light-hearted and harmless.

Client control

Control of an individual client by the peer group has a place in residential care as it does in the wider society. But in this matter, as in others, it is a question of degree. Clients should never be allowed or encouraged to exercise those forms of control which would be considered unacceptable in staff.

Corporal punishment

The use of corporal punishment with adults can never be justified. Its use as a means for punishing children in residential facilities has, however, been supported on the grounds that it is a normal feature in socialising the young. Since present trends are based upon the normalisation principle, it is argued that it would be abnormal to exclude it. Its use has

also been supported by the suggestion that it is an immediate and just way of dealing with unacceptable behaviour, and far better than forms of punishment based on emotional manipulation. While there is some validity in these arguments, there are probably stronger reasons for the exclusion of corporal punishment as an acceptable form of response in residential care. In general, it should be seen as unacceptable for children because:

its meaning in the context of residential care is different from that in a child's own home

There are considerable differences in the meaning of corporal punishment when administered by parents to their children and by employees of organisations to other people's children. The fact that staff have a role in relation to a child which is different from that of a parent is in itself sufficient to suggest the inappropriateness of corporal punishment. It is also the case that parents are likely to use it more appropriately and effectively. In the parental situation corporal punishment is administered in the context of intimate, committed and long-term relationships — dimensions which are not normal features of residential situations. Finally, and perhaps most significantly, many western societies now view corporal punishment, with some exceptions such as that which takes place in the context of the parent–child relationship, as a form of abuse.

administering corporal punishment is often irrational

While, in theory, corporal punishment should be administered rationally as a response to unacceptable behaviour, in practice its use more often than not relates to the mood of the adult. As a result, there is usually little consistency in its application. A particular action on the part of a child can elicit varying responses from adults according to their feelings at the time — one day it may be a smack, another an amused smile. While this may be acceptable and probably does little harm in the context of the parent–child relationship, it should not be seen as acceptable in residential care. Staff employed as carers have an obligation to find consistent and humane ways of responding to unacceptable behaviour without resorting to outbursts involving corporal punishment.

violence breeds violence

Helpers resorting to violence as a form of control tend to create situations where their colleagues have to behave in similar ways. Violence then becomes the standard for obtaining compliance. Since the behaviour of clients often mirrors that of staff, the more staff resort to violence the more clients are likely to do so.

Thus, punching, smacking, shaking, pinching, squeezing, biting or any other action on the part of staff that inflicts physical pain on a client should be seen as unacceptable.

CONCLUDING REMARKS

It should be recognised that a successful residence is not one where difficulties and problems are absent. Indeed, to strive for their absence is to fail to understand the realities of close and intimate living. Conflict, disagreement and mood change characterise the daily lives of people living together and should be seen as normal in a residence for disabled people. Perhaps, however, a successful residence can be identified in terms of the extent to which gross forms of unacceptable and abnormal behaviour are absent and the ability of the total group to deal effectively with its problems. But everyday difficulties will remain, and as clients gain greater control of their lives and become free of staff dominance, new kinds of problems are likely to arise.

PART | # FOUR

Managing residential services

PART FOUR

Managing residential
services

Although almost all assistance to disabled people is provided within organisational contexts, the implications of this fact for the quality of service provision are rarely appreciated. Whatever helpers strive to achieve for clients on an individual basis, a broad range of organisational factors influence and intrude upon what they do. Since most helpers, including those in senior positions, have little awareness of these factors, their analysis of and responses to situations and events often miss the reality of what is happening.

The wealth of literature on organisations confirms the significance of organisational and managerial dimensions in the attainment of goals. Managerial styles of those in senior positions, in particular, are crucial in shaping the experiences and behaviour of workers. In helping organisations there is evidence to suggest that the way managers deal with helpers shapes the way helpers deal with clients. An analysis of the present mode of operation of many helping organisations suggests the typical managerial style to be directive or authoritarian, and one that is incapable of delivering services that are consistent with the more enlightened goals now sought for disabled people. If the humane and caring objectives those in senior positions set for themselves and staff are genuine, and not empty rhetoric, it is essential that they adopt a managerial style that is consistent with these objectives.

The aims of this fourth part are to offer a range of ideas from which all levels of worker can understand what is happening in residential contexts on an organisational level, and to provide practical suggestions to enable managers to improve the ways in which they deal with workers and organisational issues. Chapter 17 lays a foundation for discussion in later chapters by considering the qualities and skills desired of all who are involved in assisting disabled people. Chapter 18 looks specifically at the role of the manager, and suggests an appropriate management style for residential organisations. Chapter 19 applies the ideas of Chapter 18 to a number of the more important dimensions of organisational life that concern the management of staff. Chapter 20, reflecting the need for residential facilities to operate in ways that are more consistent with contemporary conceptions of disabled people, looks at organisational change and ways of achieving it. Chapter 21 explores three important aspects of residential life that influence, directly or indirectly, the quality of client experiences, that is, staff training, duty rosters of direct care staff and the role and functions of boards of management. Finally, Chapter 22 discusses ways in which residential services can become more accountable for what they do.

Past and present role of the helper
Major dimensions of the helper role
Personal characteristics of the effective helper

17

The effective helper

As a foundation for the discussions in the following chapters on managing residential facilities, this first chapter explores the role and personal attributes of helpers assisting disabled people. While the skills required of helpers will vary according to position and responsibilities, it remains the case that the personal qualities desired of them will not differ greatly whatever their level of appointment.

PAST AND PRESENT ROLE OF THE HELPER

The approaches helpers take in responding to disabled people are shaped by the society of which they are members. Where that society is subject to continual change, as has been the case in western societies over the past two hundred years, the approaches of helpers will also change. In looking at some of the changes in western societies as they relate to disabled people, it is evident that the most significant developments have taken place in the past twenty years. Today, in contrast to the situation prevailing at the beginning of the 1970s, it is clear that disabled people are perceived in a quite different way. This new way of regarding them has major implications for the helping task, and this brief section contrasts the nature of the helper role as defined in the past with that of today.

In the past, disabled people were numbered amongst society's deviant groups. The major

173

reason why this was so related to the narrow and limiting conception of normality on which social life was based, and the consequent intolerance of, and hostility towards, those who differed from others. While approaches to many deviant groups were cloaked in the language and sentiment of concern, they actually served to affirm conceptions of deviance and consequently were not in the best interests of the individuals concerned. This negative evaluation of people perceived as deviant led to the development of groups of workers responsible for managing them on society's behalf. These workers were given considerable power and authority to accomplish their task, and the professional posture they adopted was not unlike that of the medical practitioner in that they assumed themselves to be expert and to know what was best for their charges. Their sense of expertise was reinforced by dogmatic and simplistic notions of clients and their needs, by attitudes of superiority and expectations of client deference. Clients and their families were usually excluded from decision-making about themselves, and those who attempted to exert influence were, more often than not, put in their place by 'we know best' responses. Since the actions of helpers tended to be justified in terms of humanitarianism, philanthropy and charity, clients had little alternative but to accept what was done to them and be grateful.

Today's approaches are based on a much broader definition of normality, one that does not perceive variations in physical and intellectual capability as denoting abnormality. As a result, approaches to disabled people are no longer built upon conceptions of difference, inferiority and unacceptability but normality and equality. The person who happens to be disabled is not seen as qualitatively different from other members of society but as equal to them, and therefore entitled to the same rights and freedoms. When this approach is applied to the behaviour of helpers it means that not only are they expected to ensure that clients have control of their lives but that they make themselves accountable to clients for their actions.

MAJOR DIMENSIONS OF THE HELPER ROLE

The major dimensions of the helper role in the residential setting are:

> *Helper and clients in partnership*
> *Helper as advocate*
> *Helper as key worker*
> *Helper as team member.*

Helpers and clients in partnership

A helping relationship should be based on the notion of partnership between helper and client, that is, a relationship where there are no status differences or elements of superiority and inferiority but equality, reciprocity, mutual support and co-operation.

Responsibility for taking the first steps in establishing a helping relationship rests with helpers and this they can do by presenting themselves as caring and concerned people. In the way they relate they should be warm, trusting, considerate, open and attractive. Effective helping relationships can never be established where helpers are experienced as distant and disinterested.

In establishing the right kinds of relationships helpers will need to:

- acknowledge their accountability to clients
- respect clients as individuals and recognise their right to independence, choice and self-determination
- remain sensitive to the needs, moods and feelings of clients
- involve clients in all decisions likely to affect them
- ensure that clients are never compelled to do that which is either against their wishes, exploitative or abnormal
- be aware of the impact and consequences of their efforts to help.

Establishing and maintaining effective helping relationships is often far from easy. The fact that workers are paid to help and that other helpers comprise their reference group often makes their interests and goals quite different from those of clients. Furthermore, the organisations within which they seek to assist clients frequently create pressures and difficulties which undermine the establishment and maintenance of effective helping relationships.

Helper as advocate

An integral aspect of the helper role is that of advocate. Workers today are expected to represent the interests of clients with whom they work to ensure they receive all services they need. The advocate dimension of the helper role involves:

- becoming fully aware of individual clients and their needs
- providing clients with information about themselves and the services to which they are entitled
- actively participating in the development of client plans
- ensuring that decisions made at client planning meetings are acted upon
- responding to and taking action on client complaints
- criticising inadequate conditions in residences and unacceptable behaviour of colleagues
- enabling clients to develop skills to act on their own behalf.

The success of the helper as advocate is dependent upon, firstly, qualities and skills such as commitment to clients, the ability to act responsibly and professional credibility. Secondly, it is closely related to the maturity of the organisation in which the helper works, particularly in terms of the way in which it deals with helper comment, criticism and complaint on behalf of clients.

Helper as key worker

A key worker is an individual who accepts responsibility for ensuring that a particular client receives all forms of assistance detailed in an individual plan, and provides personalised assistance to that client. The idea of helper as key worker, like that of helper as advocate, is quite new. Its development reflects certain deficiencies in past approaches, particularly:

- an inflexible and depersonalised approach to disabled people as a result of the belief that all within a particular category of disability had identical needs
- the existence of rigid boundaries and minimal co-operation between professional workers resulting in no unified conception of a client's overall needs and unco-ordinated efforts to help.

The key worker for each client will be the individual who has most contact with or who is of most significance to a client. Where a key worker is to be a helper, the position that person occupies in the organisation should not be of relevance. The person selected will, however, possess or be helped to acquire all necessary skills to work effectively on behalf of a client.

Among the concerns and responsibilities of key workers are:

- involvement in intake decisions, including any preliminary work with clients and families
- pre-reception arrangements
- participation in all client planning meetings
- ensuring that recommendations of planning meetings are implemented
- maintenance of client records
- provision of specific programs for clients
- maintenance of contacts with relatives of clients
- involvement in the purchase and care of a client's clothing and other personal possessions where the client requires such assistance
- acting as advocate for a client.

Helper as team member

In almost all helping contexts the task of meeting the needs of clients is one that is pursued within the context of a team. It is essential that individual workers understand what teamwork involves, particularly in terms of its consequences for the way they personally behave. So often in the past the tasks of helpers have been defined without reference to the teamwork dimension, not surprisingly resulting in hostility among and competition between workers.

To become effective team members, individual workers should:

- recognise the interdependence that exists between themselves and colleagues
- develop personal ways of behaving that are helpful to others
- continually evaluate their own performance in terms of its impact on others
- develop personal attributes, such as honesty, tactfulness and receptivity to personal criticism
- develop skills to avoid unnecessary conflicts with colleagues and to resolve them when they occur
- recognise and appreciate the skills and qualities of colleagues and the differing ways in which they are of value to clients.

PERSONAL CHARACTERISTICS OF THE EFFECTIVE HELPER

Effective helpers can be defined as:

> *Individuals who have developed appropriate and consistent sets of attitudes, beliefs and standards, and acquired necessary knowledge and skills to assist disabled people in ways they wish to be assisted, and in a manner consistent with their rights as members of society.*

Among the qualities, understandings and skills essential for effective helping are:

> *Self-understanding*
> *Commitment to clients*
> *Knowledge of client need*
> *Helping skills*
> *Awareness of work environment.*

Self-understanding

It is almost impossible to be an effective helper without considerable self-understanding and consequent self-management.

This can be developed through a process of self-evaluation by asking such questions as:

- What are my motives for undertaking this work?
- Do I have sufficient knowledge of disabled people and their needs?
- Do I have adequate skills?
- How do I present myself so that I am experienced as a caring person?
- What are colleagues and clients communicating to me about my impact on them and the way in which I do my job?
- To what extent do I expect conformity, dependence and a sense of gratitude from clients?

Self-awareness is not something that is attained at a particular point in time, it is a continuous process, with understandings and perceptions building upon or replacing others. Furthermore, since a helper's life, like that of anyone else, is never static, changes outside work need to be understood in terms of their consequences for work performance.

Commitment to clients

A strong sense of commitment to clients is a prerequisite for effective helping. It is important for a helper, not merely to be aware of this commitment on a feeling level, but to demonstrate and communicate it to clients through obvious concern, interest and respect.

A high degree of personal commitment leads to a pattern of behaviour which structures not only the way in which helpers approach and respond to the needs of clients, it actually becomes an integral dimension of their self-concept, leading to a strong sense of responsibility. Thus, committed workers set high standards for themselves which include:

- recognition that employment can be justified only in terms of real assistance given to clients
- acceptance of responsibility for personal actions. Irrespective of the behaviour of colleagues or more senior workers, the committed worker will accept total respon-

sibility for his/her actions

- acknowledgement that effective helping involves obligations to colleagues as well as to clients

Knowledge of client need

Disabled people cannot be assisted unless helpers have extensive knowledge of their backgrounds and needs. This body of knowledge includes an understanding of:

- past approaches to disabled people and the way they continue to undermine contemporary approaches
- contemporary approaches, together with the beliefs on which they are based
- limitations experienced by disabled people as a result of personal disability and the handicapping nature of social life
- necessary personal and interpersonal skills needed by clients to be able to function as effectively as possible in mainstream society.

Helping skills

To be able to assist disabled people helpers should develop a wide range of skills relating to:

- establishing helping relationships
- evaluating a client's life situation and needs
- developing client plans
- devising and implementing specific programs to meet need
- helping to resolve client problems
- integrating clients into mainstream society
- creating living environments which are normal and of benefit to clients.

Awareness of work environment

Of particular relevance to effective helping is an awareness of the working environment in terms of its impact on the helping process. This awareness includes an understanding of:

- the nature of organisations and their typical structures
- the ways in which the traditions of organisations give rise to certain courses of action and inhibit others
- the structures, characteristics and mode of operation of the particular organisations of which helpers are members
- the responsibilities and expertise of other workers within an organisation.

18

Effective management in the residential context

Of the many factors affecting client experiences in residential settings, one of the most significant, yet also the most overlooked, is the management dimension. There is considerable evidence to indicate that the way managers treat direct care workers shapes the way they treat clients. Where direct care staff experience those in senior positions as positive, helpful and caring there is every likelihood they will treat clients as they themselves are treated. Where, on the other hand, relationships between managers and carers are hostile and unhelpful, these negative dimensions are almost bound to be reflected in direct care worker–client relationships.

In exploring the management task in residential settings, this chapter seeks to clarify both the basic understandings on which good managerial practice should be based and the managerial style most likely to be effective. The two chapters that follow apply these ideas to several areas of organisational life for which managers have responsibility.

THE MANAGEMENT TASK

A manager can be defined as:

> *A person occupying a formally designated role in a work organisation which involves responsibility for the work of others.*

Thus individuals who are responsible for one, two, five, ten or a hundred workers are all managers although, of course, their power, responsibilities and skills will vary with position.

The management task essentially entails the effective use of staff in pursuit of an organisation's goals. It follows that in residential settings, as in other organisational contexts, managers cannot actually attain those goals directly as a result of their own efforts. Furthermore, the greater their seniority, and the more removed they are from the actual helping task, the more significant become their skills in attaining the organisation's goals through others.

Since management is about enabling workers to be effective, any evaluation of the performance of managers should be related to the performance of the staff for whom they are responsible. Where managers themselves are looking for evidence of their competence, they should explore the functioning of staff in relation to their own behaviour.

Factors affecting the management task

The manner in which managers relate to workers and deal with organisational issues is shaped by many factors both external to and within the organisations of which they are members. Recognising these factors and appreciating their significance are essential elements of good managerial practice. Where the understanding of managers is inadequate, they will remain incapable of solving many of the problems confronting them. Not only does this contribute to a pattern of life where things never seem to get better, it creates a sense of failure in managers which is often coped with by denying the existence of problems so obvious to others.

The following two sections attempt to provide a basis for understanding the operation of residential organisations today by exploring relevant social trends and historical factors.

SOCIAL TRENDS AFFECTING MANAGEMENT

The nature of organisational life has been undergoing considerable change in recent years, mainly as a consequence of certain social trends. Among such trends managers should appreciate are:

> *Decline in traditional forms of authority*
> *Challenge to the work ethic*
> *Demand for job satisfaction.*

Decline in traditional forms of authority

Until quite recently, a common belief in western societies was that seniority in position, higher socio-economic status, formal qualifications, greater age or being male automatically conferred authority. Over the past twenty years a trend away from this belief has been evident, and has reached the point today where many people no longer accept the directives of, or defer to, those in traditional authority positions.

This decline in ascribed authority means that the previously accepted ways of dealing with workers in organisations are now under challenge. It is fairly common today to find workers who consider it normal and appropriate to question the decisions and directives of those in more senior positions, and believe their views on issues to be equally as important as those of others. This general trend is part of the movement towards greater organisational democracy and has already undermined the manager's assumed right to issue directives without question.

Challenge to the work ethic

The importance of work, both to society and to the individual, is under challenge at the present time. This is because of:

- financial support for those unable or unwilling to work
- a decline in occupation as a measure of status and self-worth
- considerable job security, irrespective of competence.

As a result of such factors, the attitudes of people to and at work are quite different from those of only a few years ago. No longer is work valued to the extent it once was and no longer is the threat of dismissal sufficient to motivate. Organisations today find themselves in a position where they have to function quite differently than was the case in the past to attract, motivate and retain staff.

Demand for job satisfaction

Many organisations, expecially those assisting disadvantaged people, attract workers who expect to gain a great deal personally from work. They are not motivated by a desire simply to exchange time and energy for an income but have a need to attain satisfaction from what they do. This pursuit of job satisfaction is accompanied by a high personal commitment to the helping task, an expectation of involvement in decision-making and, in the context of residential care, a desire to be of significance in the lives of clients.

HISTORICAL FACTORS AFFECTING RESIDENTIAL ORGANISATIONS

The provision of services for disabled people in residential contexts takes place within formal organisations. While this is self-evident, it is a fact that needs emphasising because it helps to make sense of much activity which appears to have little to do with client need. There is a tendency, in residential as in other organisational contexts, for practices and traditions to evolve which, quite irrespective of their real value, become the realities and constraints around which life is organised. Of the many factors within residential organisations which affect the quality of help, and which managers should recognise and deal with if services are to improve, are:

> *Counter-productive organisational structures*
> *Shared negative definitions of clients*
> *Organisational stability as a barrier to change.*

Counter-productive organisational structures

Most residential facilities go back many years. At the time they came into being it was normal for organisations to be tightly structured and controlled, and it was not surprising that residential services took on this mode of operation without questioning its relevance to their overall task. As it happened, it was not entirely unsuitable in that it was consistent with the original task of residential services which emphasised client containment and control.

While approaches to disabled people have undergone major change in recent years, there has been little real change in the structures of organisations assisting them. As a result, although many managers are committed to more enlightened approaches, they are attempting to achieve change within structures that negate their basic objectives. As the discussion later in this chapter asserts, the process by which helping organisations assist clients must be consistent with the goals they are seeking to attain. In other words, the ends sought are dependent upon the means used.

Shared negative definitions of clients

The beliefs about disabled people which led to an emphasis on control and containment also emphasised incompetence. People with physical or intellectual disabilities — and the two groups were often confused — were seen as inadequate and incapable of developing basic personal and social skills. Beliefs of this kind dominated thinking in residential settings, and in many situations are still vigorously supported.

Whatever the nature of collective definitions, they tend to be communicated to new workers through the process of worker socialisation. In having little or no knowledge against which to evaluate what is communicated, new workers are understandably influenced by the shared views of more experienced colleagues and inevitably adopt collective definitions and beliefs without question. Trained workers are sometimes no less likely than others to be influenced in this way. Where such collective definitions are built around conceptions of client incompetence, change based on more enlightened beliefs has little chance of succeeding.

Organisational stability as a barrier to change

Organisations cannot function without considerable stability, and this is achieved through structure and rules. The cost of stability, however, is considerable in that it creates rigidity both in organisational processes and worker behaviour, and opposition to all forms of change. As a result, practices and procedures of long ago continue to be favoured even when they are entirely inappropriate because they are felt to be essential to the life and survival of the organisation.

EFFECTIVE MANAGEMENT

As a result of an awareness that managers develop fairly set and consistent ways of dealing with organisational issues and with staff, discussions about management behaviour tend to focus on management styles. Not only is this orientation useful in making sense of the attitudes and behaviour of managers, it enables the relationship between the behaviour of managers and workers to be explored. One of the most significant outcomes of this line of enquiry is the realisation that much worker behaviour is a consequence of managerial behaviour. This makes it possible to assert, and quite contrary to the more usual beliefs about what determines worker competence, that the performance of workers is not so much a consequence of the attitudes, knowledge and skills they bring to their jobs but an outcome of the ways in which they are managed.

It should be borne in mind that while the notion of management style is useful in understanding management behaviour and the functioning of staff, it is at the same time somewhat limited because it tends to oversimplify quite complex processes. In reality, not only are there as many styles as managers, each manager tends to use variations in style according to problems and issues being dealt with. Yet while that is so, the existence of patterning in managerial behaviour is obvious, and the concept of management style significant in understanding the behaviour of managers and the functioning of organisations.

What are management styles?

As the above discussion indicates, a management style is the consistent way in which a manager deals with staff and responds to organisational issues. While the literature on this topic explores management styles in a variety of ways, perhaps the most useful approach from the point of view of helping organisations is to seek an understanding by means of the contrasting styles of directive and participative management.

Directive management

The behaviour of the directive manager is built upon an assumption that managers have both a right and a duty to instruct staff as to how they should undertake work assigned them, and that workers, as a condition of being employed, are obliged to comply with those instructions.

This basic orientation to the management task results in a style where managers:

- retain all power belonging to their positions
- make decisions without consulting those likely to be affected by them
- are formal in dealings with staff
- restrict communications to directives and requests
- insist on conformity, and value staff in terms of complaince
- believe close supervision of staff to be essential.

Some writers consider this style to be appropriate in organisations where the tasks of workers can be clearly prescribed, where little or no discretion is required and where staff have no expectations of job satisfaction. In view, however, of the increasing hostility to authoritarianism in contemporary society, directive styles of management may become untenable in all organisations. In any event, the research on this topic suggests there to be more disadvantages than advantages associated with directive management in that it:

- results in low worker commitment
- prevents workers attaining job satisfaction
- leads to feelings of alienation
- leads to low morale, absenteeism, stress and high staff turnover
- inhibits the exercise of discretion and initiative
- results in rigid attitudes and inflexible work practices.

Participative management

In contrast to directive management, this style reflects the belief that attaining the goals of an organisation is dependent upon the involvement of staff in decision-making, and the delegation to them of considerable responsibility. This belief leads to a pattern of behaviour where managers:

- actively seek to delegate
- involve staff in all decision-making processes where the outcome is likely to affect them
- relate informally to them
- encourage open and two-way communication
- view themselves equally accountable to workers as workers are to them
- encourage the generation of ideas which differ from their own.

Participative managers operating effectively are able to create positive organisational climates where:

- staff are committed to what they are doing
- staff are able to experience considerable job satisfaction
- standards of work are high
- relationship between levels of staff are harmonious.

Is participative management always better?

The above discussion clearly suggests participative forms of management to be more effective than directive forms. While this may increasingly become the case in the future, it is important to appreciate that in reality the two styles are extremes of a continuum and that there are varying degrees of participative and directive management. Thus is is not a question of managers having to adopt one of these two extremes in styles in their entirety. Two important factors managers should consider when establishing their own management styles are:

- the relationship between management practices and the task of the organisation. There should be considerable congruence between the two and so, for example, the most appropriate style for managing a prison cannot be the same as that for running a voluntary meals on wheels service
- consistency between management practice and the stage of development of an organisation. Factors such as an organisation's history, traditions and expectations should be taken into account. Even where a change from directive to participative management is desirable, too rapid a change can sometimes worsen rather than improve a situation.

MANAGEMENT STYLES AND RESIDENTIAL CARE

In general, management styles which maximise participation of staff are more likely to be successful in residential care because:

- the quality of client life is related to the behaviour of direct care workers, and their performance is, in turn, dependent upon the way they are treated by senior staff. In short, managers communicate by their actions a style of caring other staff use in their dealings with clients

- management of staff should be consistent with philosophies governing help to clients. Since contemporary approaches emphasise client independence, personal responsibility and involvement in decision-making it would be unreasonable to expect staff to respond to quite contrary principles
- services for disabled people are experiencing considerable pressure for change. To ensure that appropriate change takes place helpers should be managed in ways that not only encourage them to be receptive to new ideas but which involve them in all stages of change processes
- stress appears at the present time to be an inevitable feature of work with disabled people. Managers should behave in ways which both minimise its occurrence and enable them to deal with it when it does occur
- providing high quality services necessitates teamwork and this can only be attained when managers are perceived and experienced by staff as important and valuable team members
- most people in helping roles, including voluntary workers, are seeking a sense of personal achievement and satisfaction from what they do. Evidence suggests this to be dependent upon the ways in which they are managed.

In summary, participative management is better suited to the management of residential services, since workers enjoying high levels of participation display or experience:

- high job satisfaction
- considerable self-worth
- positive relationships with managers and colleagues
- a willingness to accept responsibility
- a high level of commitment to their employing organisation and its goals
- a keeness to acquire greater knowledge to enable them to be more effective helpers
- positive feelings about their future
- an ability to cope with change.

Developing a personal management style

In seeking to develop a management style suited to the task of residential care, managers should first explore the beliefs on which they base their managerial behaviour. At the outset it is necessary to acknowledge certain facts about management, that is:

- it is a skill that, like other skills, can be learned
- it is essentially about dealing with the realities of organisational life rather than defining what ought to be
- it is the key dimension that determines the day-to-day effectiveness of an organisation
- the beliefs of managers generally shape the way they deal with and relate to workers. In other words, their beliefs are inclined to become self-fulfilling prophesies.

When examining their own performance managers should explore:

- what they are seeking to accomplish and the general style they are using to do so
- the nature of their behaviour and its impact on others
- the degree of consistency between their personal style, the goals of the organisation and the styles of other managers
- the beliefs and assumptions on which their dealings with staff are based
- the reasons they tend to use to explain their own and their workers' failures
- their own code of professional behaviour.

Information on effective management suggests good managers:

- as people
  — are competent, confident and reliable
  — display pleasing personal qualities such as courtesy, fairness, helpfulness and integrity
  — do not grant themselves liberties they deny to others, that is, they do not put themselves above agreements, policies and rules
  — stand by their convictions
  — are good organisers

— are aware of the impact they have on others
— accept criticism of their own performance.
- as decision makers:
  — involve others in decisions likely to affect them
  — work at the pace of staff when implementing decisions
  — accept responsibility for decisions.
- in relating to workers:
  — demonstrate genuine interest and concern
  — appreciate problems from their perspective

— treat them as individuals rather than as identical members of a group
— recognise, use and develop individual skills
— provide opportunities for self-direction and growth
— acknowledge good work
— do not expect them to do what they themselves would not do
— do not avoid commenting critically on their performance, but do so in constructive ways.

19

Practical aspects of management

This chapter explores a number of the more important areas of residential life where the functioning of managers is significant in determining both the general work atmosphere and the performance of staff. The areas considered are:

Conditions of service
Recruitment and selection
Induction
Staff support
Teamwork
Decision-making
Manager–worker communication
Meetings
Stress
Problem workers.

CONDITIONS OF SERVICE

Senior managers are responsible for establishing conditions of service and operational policies for staff including:

- appointment details such as salary, expenses, hours of work, holiday entitlement, sick leave and periods of notice
- job descriptions
- grounds and procedure for suspension or dismissal
- details of probationary periods
- procedures by which staff can make formal complaints or express grievances
- study assistance.

This information should be available to staff on appointment and changes formally communicated as they are made.

RECRUITMENT AND SELECTION

Recruiting and selecting staff is often accorded low priority in many organisations responsible for residential accommodation and, as a result, sometimes leads to bad appointments. It is important that managers recognise this to be one of their major tasks, and one which merits appropriate input in terms of personal commitment, time and effort. Among the reasons why this should be so are that:

- opportunities to fill some positions do not occur very often and good or bad appointments can have far-reaching and long-term consequences
- workers represent considerable financial investment and so should not be appointed without a thorough selection process
- not only is it damaging to organisations to appoint unsuitable people, it is also unfair to the individuals concerned
- terminating the employment of unsuitable employees is far from easy, and the general stress that results from attempts to do so can be quite destructive to all involved
- experiences at the time of recruitment and selection can be significant in influencing the expectations and commitment of new workers
- recruitment and selection processes are also exercises in public relations. There are always more unsuccessful than successful candidates and their experiences should be no less positive than those of the person appointed. Unsuccessful candidates should be left with good impressions of the organisation, a feeling that they were treated considerately and given equal opportunity to compete for the position.

The recruitment and selection process can be broken down into a number of stages. These are:

Responding to a vacancy
Attracting applications
Short listing for interview
Planning formal selection
The formal interview
Offering the position.

The information that follows is not meant to suggest an ideal way of recruiting and selecting staff but as offering ideas which may be of some value in improving existing practices.

Responding to a vacancy

When a position becomes vacant it is an appropriate time to consider whether any changes should be made in terms of duties and responsibilities. Resolving this issue is likely to involve an appraisal of the tasks carried out by the previous employee and the functioning of others with whom that person worked. In most situations it will probably be evident that no changes are required and that the position should be filled as soon as possible.

The first step in filling a vacancy will be to attract candidates, but before actually doing so two statements should be prepared:

- *Job description*: this is a statement defining the position and includes details of responsibilities, duties, salary, hours of work and work location.
- *Worker specification*: This statement attempts to set out the characteristics required of the successful applicant and details such factors as age, experience, qualifications, skills and knowledge.

Both statements will be useful when:

- preparing advertisements
- short-listing for interview
- planning and conducting formal interviews
- deciding to whom a position should be offered.

Attracting applications

The manner in which a vacancy is advertised will vary according to:

- its importance to an organisation
- degree of difficulty likely to be encountered in attracting suitable candidates
- the amount of time those responsible for the selection process are able to give to it.

Generally, the more a position is appropriately advertised the greater the likelihood of attracting an impressive number of applications. In whatever way advertising takes place, and whatever its form, information should be included that details:

- the nature of the position, responsibilities and salary
- the manner in which applications should be made
- the name of a contact person for informal discussion
- the closing date for applications.

Short-listing for interview

Where there are many applications for a position it will be necessary to prepare a short-list for interview. This is a task that should be undertaken by those actually responsible for the appointment or who will be involved in formal interviews.

The size of a short-list will be dependent on the amount of time to be given to formal selection and the form it will take. For most positions a short list of six people will be sufficient.

Those to be invited for formal interview should be notified and encouraged to visit the residence informally beforehand. The more applicants see of a residence the more aware they will be, and the more an organisation sees candidates before they are formally interviewed the greater the likelihood of making the right appointment.

Planning formal selection

Most appointments tend to be made as a result of a single formal interview. There are a number of reasons for suggesting this to be an inadequate and unreliable way of selecting staff, for example:

- most formal interviews tend to be brief, over-structured and stressful for all concerned
- anxious interviewers tend to talk too much, so limiting the contributions candidates are able to make
- the formality of interviews sometimes enables interviewers or candidates to be deceptive or dishonest.

Contemporary personnel practice suggests that formal selection should entail more than a single interview with each candidate. There are a number of ways of extending this process, one of which has proven to be of value when selecting staff for residential care. This involves inviting all short-listed candidates to be involved in a formal selection process spread over a day. A typical program for such a day is outlined in Table 19.1.

Table 19.1 A program for the selection of residential staff

Stage One	Arrange program, wherever possible, in the setting in which the successful applicant will work. Prepare clients and staff beforehand
Stage Two	Invite candidates to arrive at the same time, welcoming them with coffee
Stage Three	Where clients do not object, show candidates the residence and make appropriate introductions
Stage Four	Meet formally with candidates to clarify personnel matters, to consider briefly the characteristics of the post to be filled and to deal with any general questions
Stage Five	Invite the candidates as a group to discuss, for about 45 minutes, a topic related to the position for which they are competing. The aims in so doing will be to: <ul><li>allow candidates to demonstrate their knowledge and interests</li><li>observe how candidates function in a group situation</li><li>allow interviewers to get to know how applicants think about issues prior to formal interviews</li><li>help the candidates to become more relaxed</li></ul>
Stage Six	Provide a light lunch so that the candidates, interviewers, clients and staff can meet in a less formal atmosphere
Stage Seven	Formally interview each candidate for about half an hour

It is necessary also to give consideration to the formal interview itself to decide:

- the composition of an interview panel. Generally, a group is more effective than an individual because it is able to reduce the biases that often occur with the single interviewer. Normally not more than four people should comprise a panel. In addition to the manager responsible for the worker appointed, the panel may be made up of individuals representing other managers, staff who will work alongside the successful candidate and clients
- who will act as chairperson. The role of chairperson is important because that person will be responsible for ensuring that interviews are conducted effectively and in line with the overall program
- the general approach to be taken, including the kinds of questions to be asked and areas of questioning on which panel members may wish to concentrate.

The formal interview

An interview has a basic structure and it is the chairperson's responsibility to ensure that it is kept to by:

- introducing candidates to the interviewing situation and to panel members if they have not already met
- settling them by means of some general introductory remarks and perhaps one or two superficial questions
- explaining how the interview will be conducted and its length
- getting the interview underway by asking more probing questions
- involving other panel members
- bringing the interview to a close.

The important part of the interview will be the questioning of candidates in a way that promotes extended answers. To ensure success the following points should be borne in mind:

- all questions should be relevant

- talking by and between panel members should be kept to a minimum
- the more effective questions are those which are broad and open-ended rather than so specific as to invite yes–no type answers. For example:
  'What did you do when you worked as a volunteer?'
  'What do you think are the major difficulties disabled people face today?
  'How did you attempt to develop the social skills of the clients you worked with?'
- answers to questions should be listened to and, where appropriate, followed with supplementary questions. This tends to make the interview more conversational and often results in answers that reveal attitudes and feelings as well as providing factual information
- questioning should be thorough. If an answer is not understood or a panel member feels dissatisfied with it, further questions should be asked. It will be these probing exchanges that will give a more accurate picture of candidates and at the same time provide them with an opportunity to make a significant impression. For example:
  'Could you tell me more about the reasons why you want to leave your present job?'
  'I found that answer most interesting. Why did you say that . . .?'
  'Can you tell me the exact nature of your duties and responsibilities when you worked at . . .?'
  'Exactly how long did that period of employment last?'
- Panel members should show respect and consideration for candidates and stressful questions without good reason should normally be avoided. A warm reassuring approach with frequent positive non-verbal responses is likely to achieve greatest success
- negative judgements about candidates or their answers should not be communicated to them

- candidates should be made aware when an interview is to be brought to a close and provided with an opportunity to ask questions of a panel
- finally, information should be given about how and when candidates will learn the outcome of the interview.

Offering the position

In situations where there are a number of good candidates, it can be quite difficult to decide to whom a position should be offered. It may be helpful to ask the following questions:

- Are any candidates over-qualified and likely to become dissatisfied and outgrow the position in a short period of time?
- How will the preferred candidate fit in with the organisation and relate to clients, colleagues and managers?
- What positives and negatives is the preferred candidate likely to bring to the organisation?
- How similar are the skills, experiences and personal qualities of the preferred candidate to the original worker specification?
- How much training will the preferred candidate need to work successfully, and is it available?

Finally, and for obvious reasons, it is to the organisation's advantage not to notify the second choice candidate of the interview's outcome until the preferred candidate has formally accepted the position.

INDUCTION

All new workers should have a period of induction to acquaint them with their new work setting and its demands. The shape of a program will vary according to:

- the level at which a person is appointed
- the size of the organisation or residence
- the responsibilities of the new employee.

Among the topics that may be included in an induction program are:

- an overview of the organisation's philosophy and goals
- information relating to the client group being assisted
- details of helping approaches used
- clarification of formal policies and procedures
- an introduction to staff and clients with whom new workers are likely to have contact
- details of where help and advice can be obtained
- the training and support new workers can expect to receive.

STAFF SUPPORT

The personal resources and skills of new workers, and particularly those appointed to direct care positions, are likely to be quite limited and so it is essential that continuous support be provided to enable them not merely to survive but to grow into capable and skilled helpers. Effective support will enable an individual to:

- share concerns and anxieties
- seek and obtain help and assistance
- gain an increasing understanding of the nature and implications of the caring task
- develop necessary skills for becoming an effective helper
- establish relationships with colleagues and clients and become aware of the importance of teamwork
- maintain commitment to the task
- cope with conflict and stress.

Providing appropriate ongoing support should be an integral aspect of residential life. Among the ways managers can make it available are:

- through regular formal and informal discussions initiated by them
- through formal training sessions
- through staff meetings

- by providing staff with specialist or consultant help.

TEAMWORK

It is almost impossible to provide high quality residential services if helpers do not operate effectively in teams. Surprisingly though it may seem, teamwork is not emphasised in many residential settings, and as a result individual workers tend to go their own way and disregard or remain unaware of the consequences of their behaviour for others.

Among the reasons why teamwork is so important in residential care are:

- the task of caring for a group of disabled people in a residence is shared between a number of workers
- the range of client needs are such that they cannot be met by individual workers acting alone
- what individual workers are able to achieve is dependent upon attitudes and behaviour of colleagues
- helping and caring requires consistency and continuity
- the quality of client life is shaped by the nature of interaction processes among all people in a residence, especially those between workers.

What is teamwork?

Teamwork can be defined as:

> *effective collaboration between members of a group to achieve those goals which individuals cannot achieve when acting alone.*

A team working successfully will be characterised by:

- informal and relaxed relationships
- regular discussion and open expression of opinions and feelings
- effective resolution of differences
- variation in leadership according to task

- extensive sharing of knowledge, information and ideas
- a common understanding of what the team is trying to accomplish
- decision-making based on consensus
- a network of supportive relationships
- team assessment of its own performance
- keeping to the formal task.

Developing and maintaining teams: leader responsibilities

Developing effective teamwork is the responsibility of formal leaders, but once teams have acquired lives of their own, maintenance will be the responsibility of all members. The general approach of formal leaders in developing teams should be consistent with the participative style of management considered in the previous chapter. The areas for which formal leaders should always assume some personal responsibility are:

> *Understanding impact of own performance*
> *Enabling team members to appreciate their impact on each other*
> *Developing and using the skills of members*
> *Evaluating team performance*
> *Keeping a team to its task*
> *Resolving difficulties and dealing with conflict.*

Understanding own performance

The manner in which a formal leader relates to a team and to individual members will serve as a model for the way members relate to him/her, to each other and to clients. Effective teamwork is therefore dependent upon the personal example of the formal leader. Among the skills and understandings formal leaders should demonstrate to team members are:

- the ability to understand issues from the point of view of team members
- effectively relating to team members and others beyond the team

- openness and non-defensive reactions to criticisms of their own performance
- competence in managing informal discussions and leading meetings.

Impact of team members on each other

The formal leader will need to work both at the group and individual level to help members appreciate that:

- there are, and always will be, differences in beliefs, attitudes and skills of members
- their personal success is dependent upon the success of the team
- teamwork is essentially about co-operation
- whenever they act in ways that run counter to what has been decided by the team the consequences will almost always be detrimental
- their own beliefs and behaviour should be sufficiently flexible to accommodate changes agreed by the team.

Developing and using the skills of members

The abilities of team members vary considerably. There will be differences, for example, in skills, training, experience, commitment and aspirations. Formal leaders should recognise these differences in order to individualise the manner in which they provide support. Their efforts should focus on enabling workers to:

- extend present skills and develop new ones
- understand what others are able or wish to contribute
- use their skills to complement the work of one another
- understand the differing views others may have on the overall task.

Evaluating team performance

A formal leader can evaluate the functioning of a team by considering the:

- attainment of goals
- performance of individual members

- consequence of a team's functioning for individual members
- impact of a team on others within and beyond an organisation.

Keeping a team to its task

There will be occasions when a team will become diverted from its primary task and at such times the formal leader should assume the responsibility for helping members regain an appropriate focus.

Resolving difficulties and dealing with conflict

Any team of workers is bound to experience periods of difficulty and conflict, both at an individual and group level. These should not be viewed as detrimental, for the most part they will be looked back upon as having stimulated new ideas and growth. The presence of difficulties and conflict is indicative of a poor team only where they cannot be dealt with effectively.

The task of a formal leader will be to develop the skills of members to enable them to manage periods of stress in a way that has positive consequences. This will involve work with the team as a whole as well as with individual members.

DECISION-MAKING

The ways in which decisions are made in organisations considerably influence worker commitment, performance and morale. Evidence suggests that decision-making is most effective where it is participative, that is, where workers contribute to all decisions likely to affect them. Among the reasons why this should be so are that:

- workers are more likely to be committed to decisions they have helped to make
- better decisions are usually made as a result of group input. Ideas and information produced by a group, as well as solutions

to problems, are usually far superior to those of formal leaders acting alone

- teams working together to make decisions develop creative ways of operating that have positive consequences for other dimensions of organisational life
- a sense of involvement, open expression of views and reduction in status differences generated by participative decision-making create a climate for personal commitment and co-operation.

Actual processes for making decisions will vary according to the issues in question and the level and skills of staff involved. Decisions can be made:

- on a simple majority basis, with all workers, irrespective of position, having one vote
- through processes of consultation, that is, issues are discussed at formal and informal levels and the decision made by relevant managers. Decisions actually made will not necessarily reflect the majority view since managers may either be aware of factors not appreciated by the group or evaluate issues differently. Whatever they decide should be communicated to the workers involved together with an explanation of each decision and reasons why it was made
- by consensus, that is, unanimous agreement to a decision and support of it when operationalised despite personal reservations.

MANAGER–WORKER COMMUNICATION

Many of the problems arising in organisations assisting disabled people are related to failures in communication between senior and junior staff. This section does not attempt to explore in any detail why this should be so but seeks primarily to offer some practical suggestions to enable managers to communicate formal messages more effectively.

Managers communicate with staff verbally and in written form. Where their messages are directives, there is often an assumption that the message is necessary and the communi-

cation clear. Rarely is a directive questioned by managers in terms of possible ambiguity, problems it may cause, unfavourable reactions it may provoke or the necessity for making it in the first place. As a result, such directives are often misunderstood, ignored or responded to in a hostile way, with negative consequences for the relationship between sender and receiver.

Written versus verbal communication

If the formal messages of managers are to be effective, they should be communicated in the most appropriate way. There has been a tendency among many managers to over-use written communications because they believe them to be more effective. In reality this is not the case and unless it is impossible to speak to staff, or the communication so important that it should be circulated in written form, verbal communication is to be preferred.

Among the reasons why written communications are problematic are that they:

- often go unread. Sending a note to staff in no way guarantees it will be read. To assume it will be, when often it is not, is a failure on the manager's part to face reality
- are often misunderstood. No matter how clear communications sometimes appear to be, they can be misunderstood, particularly if receivers are hostile to the message or its sender
- can expose the sender to criticism, for example, in terms of quality of English, choice of words or attitudes implicit in the message
- can, if they are poor communications, be remembered, retained and used against the sender
- can be interpreted as a way of avoiding face-to-face confrontation. Where, for example, a written communication is intended as a criticism of one or more workers, it can be seen as a coward's way out
- create and sustain distance which negatively affects manager–worker relationships.

Spoken communications, on the other hand, can be very effective when they are well used because the communicator:

- operates from an understanding that communication is essentially a two-way process
- is in a position to know the message is received
- is able to observe reactions of receivers and respond to them
- can communicate in a considerate and caring way
- can establish patterns of communication which improve interactions with staff.

Improving written communication

Where written communications are essential, managers should ensure that:

- they write and rewrite a message until it is clear and to the point
- they comprehend a message from the point of view of those who will receive it, and particularly members of staff who seem to have a tendency to misunderstand
- they seek reactions to contentious communications from a trusted colleague before circulating them
- the way they communicate on paper is consistent with their general management style. Where a manager, for example, deals in a participative way with staff on a face-to-face level, his/her written communications should not be highly directive.

If a written communication is misunderstood and provokes negative reactions, the blame lies, for the most part, with the sender. It should be examined in the light of such responses to find out in what ways it was defective, inappropriate or poorly timed.

Communication as a two-way process

A successful organisation will be characterised by open, two-way communication, from manager to staff and staff to manager. Communications from workers to their

managers should be encouraged because they achieve much that is positive, for example, they:

- provide a clear picture of what staff think and feel
- create feelings of involvement in workers
- enable workers to contribute ideas to the running of an organisation and solutions to problems
- enable managers to remain aware of problems and difficulties encountered by staff
- close gaps between levels of staff and reduce negative feelings that seem inevitably to accompany differences in status
- have positive consequences for communication between direct care workers and clients.

MEETINGS

Meeting are a regular feature in the life of most residential facilities. There are, for example, staff meetings, meetings for the preparation of client plans, meetings between clients and helpers and meetings between clients. It is essential that meetings are well run. When they are, they:

- achieve efficient and enjoyable conduct of business
- generate co-operative feelings which tend to be transferred to other situations
- enable effective decision-making to take place
- are excellent contexts for resolving problems
- provide staff and clients with a broader appreciation of complex issues
- can be ideal contexts for staff training
- generate caring attitudes.

Many workers, and particularly direct care staff, when asked for their reactions to meetings often respond by suggesting them to be too long, unnecessary, too frequent, monopolised by senior staff, highly critical and judgemental, divisive and often not particularly pleasant. Such reactions are a reflection, not so much of meetings themselves, but of the way they are run. Ideas included therefore seek to enable those responsible for running meetings to do so more effectively.

Leading meetings

This section considers formal as opposed to informal meetings, that is, meetings called by managers. Such meetings will normally be led by the manager, although for certain issues the leadership role may be set aside or passed to another person.

Since formal leaders are responsible for ensuring that meetings run effectively, their work begins before meetings take place and usually continues after they have been concluded.

An individual leading a meeting should make certain that:

- an agenda exists and is followed. The agenda should be relevant to the meeting and be made known beforehand to those attending. The leader will work to keep the meeting to the agenda by reducing time-wasting, disruption or diversion
- each person attending has an opportunity to participate. This will involve encouraging the more reticent to contribute as well as ensuring that dominant members do not monopolise discussion. A meeting where most attending do not or cannot contribute is, for them, often unsatisfactory. If there is no need for their active participation, the necessity for the meeting should be questioned
- decisions made are in the best interests of all, particularly clients. To ensure that they are, formal leaders will need to be well acquainted with issues being discussed, various views being advanced and reasons why certain positions are taken. They will also need to be aware of the dynamics of meetings and particularly the way pressure for certain decisions builds up
- the meeting generates feelings of co-operation and positiveness. This calls for flexibility in leadership, being directive where

necessary but also allowing meetings occasionally to go where they will. It will also involve the leader in preventing the development of conflict, stress and feelings which cannot be resolved or which will have unhelpful consequences. Additionally, the formal leader will attempt to prevent individual members from having negative experiences at meetings by being particularly supportive of those who are less assertive or more vulnerable

- difficulties and disagreements are resolved before the conclusion of a meeting. Quite often, because of poor agenda planning or time management, difficulties and conflicts arise which are not resolved. This causes individuals to leave meetings with a sense of distaste and bad feeling. If contentious issues have to be raised, or if they are allowed to surface, suffcient time should be available to recover the situation before a meeting ends
- a meeting is formally terminated. This will entail drawing discussions to a close, summarising issues, indicating points of agreement and disagreement, clarifying decisions, action to be taken and determining the date of the next meeting
- problems and issues not resolved at the meeting are dealt with in some other way
- informal discussions take place after the meeting to gauge the feelings and reactions of individuals.

The agenda

There is usually a need for some kind of agenda, although if it is too formal it can stifle communication and render a meeting rigid and meaningless.

If an agenda is thought necessary:

- it should be possible for all attending the meeting to request topics to be placed on it
- the formal leader should prepare it but not include suggested items that are inappropriate or too contentious. Such action

should be explained to the person suggesting the topic and perhaps also to the meeting
- it should be circulated beforehand
- at the commencement of a meeting the leader should clarify which items are for discussion and which require decisions, and suggest the amount of time to be given to each.

Evaluating meetings

Following each meeting the leader should personally attempt to evaluate it. This can be achieved by means of the following questions:

- Did the meeting appear enjoyable and beneficial for those present?
- Who participated and who did not?
- What problems developed?
- To what extent were problems resolved?
- Did the group work together in discussion and problem-solving?
- How did I perform as a chairperson and facilitator?

STRESS

The existence of stress in organisations has been recognised only in recent years. An increasing understanding of both its causes and destructive effects is bringing about a reappraisal of organisational life and changes in the work environment. No where has stress been more strongly experienced than in residential settings, and not only can all levels of staff be subjected to it, many clients continually experience it. In thinking about responses to stress it is important to acknowledge that damaging forms of stress are not inevitable; there is much that can and should be done to reduce its occurrence and minimise its consequences.

What is stress?

Stress is a somewhat difficult concept to define but basically it describes the effects on an individual's sense of well-being, physiological state and relationships of demands with which he/she cannot cope. These demands can be:

- in the form of unreasonable expectations made by others
- a consequence of the way in which an individual perceives external factors and events
- the result of unattainable goals individuals may set for themselves.

There is a tendency to believe that all stress is harmful. If this is so then people clearly function best when it is absent. But even the most superficial analysis of life shows that this is not the case, since without a certain degree of stress growth and development are not possible. Stress, in fact, is an everyday part of life and creates the demands and pressures giving rise to change. It is fairly normal for individuals to experience frequent periods of stress which, for the most part, are not damaging because they are understood and coped with. Some people actually welcome stress or deliberately create it for themselves because they feel it enables them to be more productive.

Stress, then, can be beneficial. The point at which it becomes damaging and counter-productive is when it exceeds an individual's ability to cope. When this happens, and no help is available, its impact can be considerable. When it is experienced in extreme form, or over an extended period of time, its effects can be devastating both on a personal and interpersonal level. Often, recovery from extreme forms of stress is partial whatever the help offered.

While stress can be experienced only on an individual level, it can be common to a number of people in that groups and sometimes whole organisations can be affected by the same kinds of stress. This can occur either as a result of being subjected to similar external pressures or because of shared perceptions of experiences.

Although the discussion in this section focuses on staff stress, it is equally important to remain aware that clients also experience stress. There is often a close relationship between staff and client stress and so action to help one group will not be effective if it disregards the other.

Recognising stress

There are many indicators of helper stress and whenever they are evident they should not be misunderstood as being indicative of poor staff. Among these indicators are:

- absenteeism and poor time-keeping
- frequent minor sicknesses such as headaches, skin complaints, stomach disorders, backaches and physical exhaustion
- regular extended breaks
- high staff turnover
- psychological lassitude, for example, tiredness, apathy, depression and avoidance of clients and colleagues
- extreme cynicism
- a desire to complete tasks with the minimum number of problems and to get away from work as quickly as possible
- continual disputes with other staff and much ill-feeling
- neglect and abuse of clients.

Consequences of stress

When individual workers experience stress with which they cannot cope it can:

- produce considerable feelings of inadequacy and lead to self-abuse
- render them introverted and totally preoccupied with their own problems
- take away all motivation
- make them unstable, short-tempered and hostile to others.

When a team experiences stress with which it cannot cope:

- it is unable to focus upon and attain its primary goal
- there is much conflict among members
- members deny their interdependence
- individuals act without considering the

consequences for others, and on occasions deliberately seek to be destructive.

When an organisation experiences stress with which it cannot cope:

- services to clients are poor
- it becomes unstable and goes from crisis to crisis
- there is a high rate of staff turnover
- morale is low
- staff are hostile to one another
- the pursuit of effective coping mechanisms becomes a major goal
- distorted definitions of what is real are rigidly maintained despite evidence to the contrary.

Burn-out

Burn-out is a term that features prominently in the literature on stress. While it sounds somewhat dramatic, it is a useful concept in that it vividly describes the consequences to individuals of continuous and intense forms of stress. People said to be burnt-out have reached the point where they are physically and emotionally exhausted, and deal in a negative and destructive way with self, others and work. Where burn-out is extreme it brings individuals to the point where they are no longer able to cope with what were once manageable tasks and responsibilities, and creates a chronically disturbed emotional state. The concept of burn-out has considerable value for residential life in that it accurately describes the condition of many helpers and clients.

What causes stress in the residential context?

It is not easy to identify what causes stress in residential care. What may at first appear to be a cause can, in reality, be seen as the consequences of a more basic cause. Alternatively, cause and effect can be so interrelated that they are part of a cycle. The behaviour of clients, for example, is often said to be a cause of helper stress, but since the way clients behave is to a considerable extent a consequence of the way in they are treated by helpers, this may be so only in a few cases.

Among the dimensions of residential life that are considered to contribute to worker stress are:

> *Pressures arising from the helper role*
> *Consequences of continually giving*
> *Client behaviour*
> *Inadequate skills and resources*
> *Disillusionment*
> *Conflict with colleagues.*
> *Conflict with managers.*

Pressures arising from the helper role

- Working in isolation and without support
- long periods of intense work with little relief
- aspects of the task which assault personal dignity
- exposure to pressures when least able to cope, for example, early in the morning and late at night
- disturbance of body rhythms and family and social life as a result of shift work.

Consequences of continually giving

- Emotionally draining relationships with clients
- never experiencing a feeling of achievement or success
- the perception of few positive responses from the particular client group
- insufficient support to retain motivation.

Client behaviour

- Fear of losing control
- concern about resorting to unacceptable ways of dealing with client behaviour
- violent episodes
- intimidating and threatening behaviour
- general unpredictability of some clients
- fear of doing the wrong thing.

Inadequate skills and resources

- Lack of training

- inadequate interpersonal skills and coping mechanisms
- reluctance to seek help because of concern about the reactions of others
- inadequate physical resources.

Disillusionment

- Sense of isolation and powerlessness
- career dead end; no possibility for training or promotion
- unrealistic initial expectations about personal success and rewards
- over-simplistic beliefs about the needs of clients
- hostile attitudes towards clients as a result of a sense of failure
- little personal recognition by others.

Conflict with colleagues

- Lack of co-operation and support
- frequent disputes and arguments
- competition for client interest and affection
- preoccupation with problems within the staff group and consequent neglect of clients.

Conflict with managers

- Disagreements over importance of administrative tasks
- experiences of being treated impersonally
- lack of recognition
- little or no delegation of responsibility
- complaints from managers about what workers consider to be trivial issues
- unreasonable expectations
- conflict between expectations of managers and needs of clients.

Most of these suggested causes are in fact the outcome of a failure on the part of managers to recognise what is actually happening in residences. The relationship between inadequate management and the continued existence of destructive stress is explored in Figure 19.2.

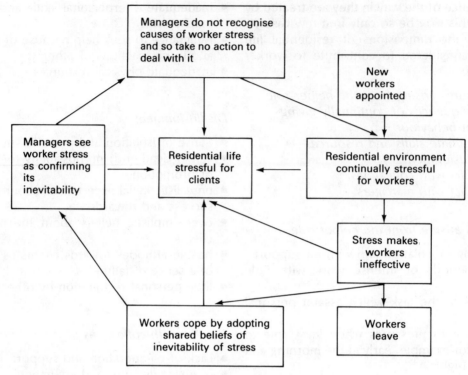

Fig. 19.1 Relationship between inadeqate management and stress.

Reducing stress

As earlier discussion suggests, there are no quick and easy ways of dealing with stress. Its reduction is dependent upon the provision of an environment and way of life which is described in this book, that is where:

- clients are able to live a normal life with all the rights and freedoms enjoyed by other members of society
- helpers function in work contexts which are totally supportive and which enable them to develop all necessary skills.

In working towards the creation of a better environment and way of life it is essential that managers take positive action to reduce worker stress. Among the skills they should develop to be able to do so are:

- recognising stress
- appreciating individual differences in:
  - tolerating stress
  - the effects of stress

- perceptions of factors and events as stressful
- coping with stress
- dealing with stress over time
- enabling individuals to become aware of stress in themselves and in others by:
  - recognising physical, psychological and interpersonal indicators of stress
  - appreciating the point at which stress becomes harmful
  - helping them to understand individual capabilities limitations
- finding practical ways of reducing stress, for example:
  - removing workers from stressful situations
  - giving time off
  - providing relevant training
  - providing opportunities to work with more skilled colleagues
  - teaching staff to anticipate and deal effectively with crises
  - teaching staff to be assertive, both to

complain when necessary and to resist the passing on of an unfair or unattainable share of the workload
— developing self-protective attitudes and behaviour
— helping staff to place their work in a realistic perspective by not expecting too much from it
— encouraging them to emotionally distance themselves from work when they are not there
— assuming responsibility for and taking action to deal with organisational factors causing stress such as insufficient numbers of staff, poor working conditions and inadequate equipment.

PROBLEM WORKERS

Problem workers are individuals whose behaviour at work is inadequate, improper or inappropriate in relation to their assigned duties and the needs and goals of the organisation. As a result of their actions they undermine the efforts of colleagues and negatively affect the quality of client care.

Once workers become a problem to others, and the more informal ways of changing their behaviour have been tried and have failed, their performance is not likely to improve without specific action on the part of the manager concerned. Failure to take action is almost bound to result in a worsening situation and a belief by others that the behaviour of the problem worker is being condoned.

Thinking about the problem worker

Before managers conclude workers to be a problem and take action, it is essential to ensure that the values against which they are making their judgements are soundly based and realistic. Where they have unrealistic ideas about the way in which organisational life should be conducted, their analysis of situations and people is unlikely to lead to the successful resolution of difficulties. Among the beliefs and values which influence the

judgements of managers and which are important to clarify are:

> *The nature of the helping task*
> *Expectations of worker competence*
> *The nature of the management task.*

Nature of the helping task

It is essential for managers to understand that just as the helping task cannot be defined in any specific way, the manner in which helpers function on a day-to-day basis cannot be tightly regulated by directives from above. The helping task is dependent upon the quality of relationships between helpers and clients and the freedom helpers are able to enjoy when responding to new and unforeseen situations. It is therefore necessary that considerable responsibility, involving the use of discretion and initiative, be delegated to workers. When it is, many differences between management expectations and worker behaviour will be an outcome of delegation, and therefore not be grounds for management criticism and complaint.

Expectations of worker competence

Many managers often appear to operate from unquestioned assumptions about the ability of workers, and react critically when incompetence is displayed. Yet the fact is that most people taking up positions in helping organisations, including recent graduates, while having a great deal of enthusiasm, are quite limited in helping skills. There is little evidence to suggest they will become effective merely with the passing of time, particularly in situations where the necessary skills are not present in their work group. Whether or not they become competent is often entirely related to the quality of assistance provided by more senior workers.

There is evidence to suggest that many workers considered by their managers to be problematic have seldom, if ever, experienced:

- a close and supportive relationship with their immediate manager
- help and support when coping with difficult situations
- feedback on their performance, so leaving them with little understanding of the way others see their efforts.

Nature of the management task

Since managers are only able to pursue the goals of organisations through the workers for whom they are responsible, it follows that they should give as much time as necessary to training and support, and to providing contexts where workers can be successful. From this perspective, workers who become problematic can be viewed, more often than not, as the outcome of inadequate management input.

Analysing problem behaviour

Before taking action to deal with problem workers, managers should ensure that their analysis of situations is accurate, and that action is both warranted and likely to attain some degree of success. This can be achieved by asking such questions as:

Why is the worker a problem?

Answering this question is likely to involve a review of:

- the actual behaviour considered unacceptable and factors relating to it
- the real as opposed to the apparent difficulties the worker is creating for others
- the kinds of interpretations being placed on the worker's behaviour
- the opinions of managers not directly responsible for the worker in question
- the worker's likely responses to criticisms of his/her behaviour
- possible factors confusing the issue, such as subjective judgments about the worker.

How damaging is the behaviour?

If it is obvious that the worker's behaviour is having serious consequences for others, be they workers or clients, the manager should take action as soon as possible but not without, of course, having planned that action.

What is action likely to achieve?

The aim in taking action will obviously be to bring about change in the attitudes or behaviour of the worker concerned. With some workers, however, goals should not be set too high as they may be capable of only quite modest change.

A proposed course of action should be explored, not only from the point of view of the worker concerned but also in relation to others involved. This kind of appraisal sometimes leads to a level of understanding that brings about a more realistic plan of action.

Action to deal with a problem worker

A manager should meet with the problem worker in the context of a formal interview to discuss the difficulties the worker appears to be causing. In aiming to bring about some improvement in the worker's behaviour the interview will try to achieve an open and frank exchange of views, a mutual understanding of the situation and agreement on action to be taken. Such interviews should be carefully planned so that the stress and conflict they tend to generate can be minimised.

The following steps may be helpful when planning such interviews:

Step one: The manager approaches the worker and arranges to meet at a mutually convenient time to discuss concerns about the worker's performance. While this is likely to create anxiety and concern in the worker and a request for clarification, an extensive discussion at this stage should be avoided.

Step two: The manager and worker meet and, in as non-threatening a way as possible, the manager explains why the worker's behaviour is considered unsatisfactory and cites evidence in support. This statement should include details only of the individual's performance at work and exclude personal factors. Since the goal of the interview will be to arrive at some positive outcome, negative criticism, as well as recounting problems from the past, should be avoided.

Step three: The worker is invited to respond to what has been said and to explain how he/she views the situation.

Step four: The manager and worker discuss what has been said and work towards an understanding that will serve as a basis for action. If the worker disagrees with the manager's analysis and nothing has been said to cause the manager to view the situation differently, the manager may consider it appropriate to let the worker know the consequences of his/her present pattern of behaviour. If such a warning is given, it should be accompanied by a statement of the worker's rights, and the worker should be given the name of a more senior person to whom he/she can appeal.

Step five: The manager concludes the interview by summarising what has been discussed, agreements reached and action to be taken. A time to meet in the near future to review the situation should arranged.

It is important when conducting such interviews to avoid confrontations and threats and to leave acceptable ways out for both parties.

If the worker's behaviour improves as a result of this process, the situation should be considered resolved and not used against the worker at any time in the future.

Unhelpful responses

Many of the more usual responses of managers to problem workers are unhelpful and tend to make situations worse. Among those that should be avoided are:

- directives such as 'Pull yourself together'
- criticism involving ridicule or sarcasm
- commands such as 'You will do exactly as I tell you'
- deliberately seeking to create fear
- hostile confrontations which simply make the worker bitter
- grumbling openly to others in the hope that they will communicate dissatisfactions to the worker concerned
- reprimanding a worker in the company of others.

Concluding comments

These ideas may not seem particularly practical when considered in relation to some of the more difficult workers who are occasionally found in residential situations. But the fact is that there can be no easy way of dealing with staff who have become extremely problematic. If good helpers are sought they should be selected carefully, trained and supported, given ongoing feedback on their performance, and provided with assistance to succeed so that they never reach the stage where they are counter-productive to an organisation and its goals.

20

The manager as innovator

As a result of the impact of contemporary thinking about the ways in which disabled people should be assisted, residential services are today experiencing considerable pressure for change. Major responsibility for responding to this pressure and instituting necessary change rests, for the most part, with workers in senior positions. In exploring change as it relates to residential services, this chapter seeks to provide managers with an understanding of some of the issues involved together with a number of practical suggestions for bringing about change.

Relatively little information exists on change, and much of what there is explores it from a theoretical perspective. This is perhaps not surprising in that, despite the fact that change has been increasing in western societies over the past two hundred years, it has until recently been viewed as something to be responded to and coped with rather than planned, anticipated and controlled. Now that change has reached the stage where it is integral to social life and is continuous, the need for a practical understanding of it is seen as an important focus of academic enquiry. At present, however, information remains quite limited, as will be reflected in the contents of this chapter.

There is, nevertheless, sufficient knowledge to assert that:

- change is continuous. While individuals, social groupings, organisations and societies may at times appear to experience periods of stability, each is, in reality, in a constant state of change. Thus, an expectation that stability can and should be attained is unnatural, and attempts to impose it are at best mistaken and at worst repressive

- change is unpredictable. While it is possible to formulate ideas for initiating change, the reality is that change processes often develop lives of their own. Even where attempts are made to tightly control change, once decisions have been taken and ideas set in motion, a wide range of factors intrude and take programs in quite unanticipated directions. As a result, a great deal of action in relation to change is about responding to and making sense of unanticipated developments
- the outcomes of programs of change are dependent upon processes used. Thus, in seeking to bring about change, those in positions to initiate it should first explore the approaches they plan to use in terms of any intended and unintended consequences.

CHANGE IN RESIDENTIAL CARE

Difficulties encountered by managers in residential settings when seeking to initiate and control change can be considerable and, and as is the case with other dimensions of the management task, it is essential to base actions on a realistic perspective of what is involved. As well as appreciating the general nature of change, a manager in a residential setting should be aware that:

- each process of change is unique
- there is no single effective way of bringing about change
- the way in which change is attempted in a particular organisation should be consistent with its general mode of operation and styles of managers involved
- individuals who initiate change become caught up in the change process and so

cannot expect to be objective about what is happening

- reactions which appear to modify a planned program of change should be viewed on their merits, rather than as necessarily undermining it
- managers do not usually achieve change. Their task is to generate ideas and create climates enabling staff involved to bring about change
- much of the change taking place in residential services today is directly or indirectly initiated by:
  — professionally trained staff, many of whom are forces for change as a result of the nature of their training
  — direct care workers
  — clients, families and pressure groups working on behalf of clients
  — legislation
  — directives from funding bodies
  — adverse publicity.

FORMULATING IDEAS FOR CHANGE

Before taking action to implement new ideas, changes sought should be explored from a number of perspectives to ensure they are appropriate, realistic and attainable. Among the questions those seeking to introduce change should ask are:

Why is change necessary?

In seeking to answer this question change should be considered in terms of:

- its consequences for clients
- its likely impact on existing ways of operating
- any questionable motives for favouring it, for example, it may be sought as a result of pressure from more senior managers or simply because a particular approach is fashionable.

Are proposals realistic?

Quite often proposals are assumed, without question, to be realistic. In order to avoid the failures that often occur when such assumptions are made it is necessary to consider:

- whether proposals are likely to work
- what is likely to happen once they are set in motion
- whether they are the most desirable proposals at that particular time
- the extent to which they are consistent with other programs of change.

What is the focus of change?

Answering this question leads to a much greater understanding of the aims of a program of change and enables its focus to become more specific. Is a program, for example, aimed at:

- staff attitudes and behaviour?
- staff skills?
- relationships between staff and clients?
- behaviour of clients?
- organisational structure and modes of operation?
- the total environment?

Who is likely to gain or lose as a result of change?

This is probably the most significant question to ask when trying to anticipate the likely reactions of others. It is neither unnatural nor surprising that those likely to benefit from change will support it, while those likely to be disadvantaged in some way will be in opposition.

What approaches have been successful in the past?

The process by which change is attempted often determines its success. Where an organisation has already achieved certain changes, it is better to use similar approaches than introduce new ones. New ways of seeking change are in themselves change processes which have to be contended with.

What is the time scale for change?

Approaches used are often dependent on the time scale involved. The quicker change needs to be achieved the more directive managers will be in their dealings with staff.

How should proposals for change be communicated?

The ways in which workers learn about proposals for change are very important. Poor or inappropriate communication can create resistance to the best ideas. In general, methods chosen should be consistent with the proposals themselves and communicated in ways most likely to elicit favourable responses. Among the ways in which ideas about change can be communicated are:

- at formal and informal meetings
- though written communications
- through an organisation's grapevine
- through individual contact.

What is the change agent's position in the organisation?

The manner in which change agents seek to achieve change should be consistent with their formal position and power within an organisation. Where they have little real power they will fail if they attempt to direct unwilling staff.

INITIATING CHANGE

There is no single correct way of achieving change in residential settings. Each situation and set of circumstances requires different approaches. The following ways of pursuing change are explored not because they are the only approaches that can be used but because consideration of them enables managers to think constructively about how they can attempt specific programs of change.

The four approaches, which have been adapted from Tannenbaum, R. and Schmidt, W. (1958) are:

> *Informing staff of change*
> *Persuading staff to accept change*
> *Consulting staff about change*
> *Participating with staff in deciding about change.*

Informing staff of change

This approach is consistent with directive managment discussed in Chapter 18. Managers inform workers of changes about to take place and do not invite them to express any opinions about what is to happen.

The advantages of this approach are:

- it has the potential to achieve change rapidly
- it suppresses objections to change which, if voiced, could undermine what is sought.

The disadvantages of this approach are:
- it can easily be sabotaged by staff opposing change
- it may achieve only short-term change
- change may need to be enforced by those in positions of authority.

Persuading staff to accept change

Managers decide what changes should be brought about and meet with staff to seek their support. In effect this approach is one where managers are attempting to sell their ideas to staff.

The advantages of this approach are:

- if staff believe that at the discussion stage they can reject a manager's proposals, they have greater feelings of involvement and power
- in being sold ideas for change, staff are more likely to be committed to them
- selling and persuading involves bargaining and negotiation and the possibility of general support for proposals.

The disadvantages of this approach are:

- acceptance of proposals is often dependent upon the skills of managers as persuaders rather than the benefits of the proposed changes
- staff can be persuaded to accept change they do not really favour and, after a time, will not support
- staff can feel manipulated and degraded.

Consulting staff about change

Managers wishing to introduce programs of change meet with staff and outline their proposals and reasons for advocating them. Their ideas are discussed by workers and managers together and modified as the group feel appropriate, but with managers retaining the power to make final decisions.

The advantages of this approach are:

- staff become fully acquainted with the reasons why change is sought and involved in the decision-making process
- ideas superior to those of managers can be suggested by staff or are developed as a result of discussion
- staff usually prefer this approach, and support its outcome even when it differs from what they personally would have preferred.

The disadvantages of this approach are:

- it enables opposition to proposals to be expressed or to be generated
- it creates a context for disagreement
- it usually involves considerable time.

Participating in decisions about change

Managers believing change to be necessary meet with staff and outline their ideas. These ideas become the starting point for discussion: staff can respond in any way they wish and modify the manager's proposals or substitute alternatives. Decisions are made by the team, the manager being one member of it.

The advantages of this approach are:

- difficulties arising from power relationships can be kept to a minimum
- ideas for change can be unanimously supported
- managers can be respected for sharing decision-making and so more attention is given to their ideas.

The disadvantages of this approach are:

- discussions about change can become dominated by a small and unrepresentative group
- managers can be seen as avoiding responsibility for decision-making
- decisions are, in retrospect, sometimes highly suspect.

Which approach is best?

While contemporary approaches to organisational decision-making suggest consultative approaches to have greatest chance of succeeding, most change programs involve many stages and are likely to require a variety of approaches. There will, in particular, be occasions when a directive approach is necessary. A point is often reached where, although verbally supporting a set of proposals, workers are at the same time reluctant to take any specific action to attain them. The step from expression of support to action sometimes needs quite firm handling on the part of the manager concerned.

A useful but by no means always practical way of considering and implementing change is outlined in Table 20.1.

THE ROLE OF THE CONSULTANT

In many situations it will be advantageous to involve consultants in analysing situations, devising change programs and implementing them. Among the benefits in using skilled consultants are:

- they often have considerable expertise in planning and implementing change

Table 20.1 A process for bringing about change

Stage 1:	Create a way of operating which encourages the generation of ideas for change
Stage 2:	Select certain ideas and encourage formal and informal discussion of them
Stage 3:	Formulate some definite proposals
Stage 4:	Discuss proposals with workers. Respond openly to all reservations and objections and modify proposals as necessary
Stage 5:	Formulate a new set of proposals and seek support from workers, particularly those holding informal leadership positions
Stage 6:	In consultation with workers, decide on a firm set of proposals
Stage 7:	Devise a plan for achieving proposals including details of what is to be done, by whom and when
Stage 8:	Implement plan and modify it as it becomes necessary
Stage 9:	Evaluate plan at an agreed future date

- in being acknowledged as experts, they have credibility which enables them to take on leadership roles
- as outsiders, they are not bound by organisational pressures and constraints and so can be more objective about what is happening and what needs to be done
- in having no formal power, they have the potential to get closer to all levels of staff
- they are people who, by their position and as result of their skills, can absorb much of the hostility to change, so diverting it from others
- they can offer fresh approaches and a range of solutions to problems
- they can take the first and often most difficult steps in initiating discussion on change and, at the appropriate moment, hand a change process to appropriate workers within an organisation.

RESISTANCE TO CHANGE

Whenever changes are proposed there is almost always some form of resistance. It is helpful to think about resistance on two levels:

Resistance at an organisational level
Resistance at an individual level.

Organisational resistance

Most organisations today are bureaucracies, that is, they have hierarchical lines of responsibilities, tasks are divided between workers and day-to-day operations are regulated by formal procedures, rules and policies. The function of a bureaucratic structure is to achieve organisational goals through a rational, stable and consistent mode of operation. While this is often attained, the cost of so doing can be rigid attitudes and practices, and the devotion of workers' energies to maintaining the status quo. In such situations, ideas for change tend to be met with negative reactions, and convincing reasons why they are unrealistic and cannot be attained.

Counteracting organisational resistance of this kind, and developing ways of operating which increase flexibility and an openness to change, should be a major focus of those in management positions. This can be achieved in a variety of ways but is essentially related to an understanding of individual resistance, even where it is within a group context.

Individual resistance

At the outset it should be realised that while workers are often hostile to new ideas, resistance is by no means always detrimental. There are often legitimate reasons for it, and so resistance should be viewed as a necessary and often integral aspect of change. Not only is it effective in highlighting defects in proposals, it also leads to tensions which generate creative and new ideas.

Resistance, then, should be considered on its merits. Those forms of it which tend to be negative are those which:

- originate in a general disposition of hostility to or fear of change
- render an individual incapable of entertaining any ideas about change
- have their origins in opposition to change as part of group loyalty.

Those forms of it which can be considered positive and as contributing to change programs are where workers:

- genuinely do not understand what is proposed and reasons why. This often arises, not merely because of poor communication or insufficient information, but because workers interpret ideas differently from managers
- earnestly believe proposals for change to be ill-conceived and wrong
- while supporting the general goals of proposals, do not believe the suggested process for attaining them to be correct
- feel they have significant ideas to contribute which would improve proposals
- may simply need more time to come to terms with what is proposed and its consequences
- see proposals as having negative consequences such as:
  — reducing their power, status and responsibilities
  — threatening their beliefs and values
  — changing their role, work situation or conditions
  — causing unreasonable stress

Responding to resistance

Among the more effective ways of responding to resistance are:

- stating as often as is necessary reasons for proposing change and likely benefits until they are understood and appreciated by all involved
- allowing time for individuals and groups to come to terms with proposals and their implications
- listening to objections, recognising those on an emotional level and accommodating and compensating for those involving genuine loss
- seeking to persuade informal leaders to support change before working with other staff
- implementing only those aspects which have general support, leaving more conten-

tious proposals until a later date

- suggesting a trial period for change, with an understanding that results will be evaluated and modified where they are felt to have been unsuccessful
- providing all necessary training to enable staff to implement and achieve changes required of them.

In general, proposals for change will succeed and resistance be minimised where managers:

- recognise the implications and consequences of change for all involved
- recognise that they themselves may need assistance in formulating and implementing ideas for change, and in coping with it as it occurs
- do not assume their ideas to be the best and only ones
- formulate proposals for change that stress benefits to clients. Staff are able to support initiatives where their sense of professionalism and desire to be of value to clients is enhanced
- avoid, whenever they can, imposing change
- support staff in adjusting to proposals

- anticipate responses and developments rather than simply react to them
- modify proposals whenever necessary but not to the point of compromising basic objectives
- develop in staff a capacity to be open and receptive to ideas for change and to take the initiative in proposing them.

REALITIES OF CHANGE

In terms of the realities of change, evidence suggests that:

- change is possible in all organisations
- many significant and necessary changes are not dependent upon an increase in finance and resources since they are essentially about attitudes, behaviour and practices
- additional resources and finance do not necessarily bring about intended changes
- change requires a disproportionate effort, commitment and determination on the part of change agents
- substantial change takes considerable time.

Staff training
Hours of direct care workers
Boards of management

21

Other management issues

This chapter explores three areas of residential life which directly or indirectly influence the quality of client experiences. They are:

> *Staff training*
> *Hours of duty of direct care staff*
> *Boards of management.*

STAFF TRAINING

Until a few years ago, with the exception of a few senior workers with nursing or clinical qualifications, helpers in residential facilities were untrained; what knowledge and skills they acquired resulted from working alongside more experienced but equally untrained colleagues. There was virtually no understanding that this way of operating imposed major limitations on the quality of help given to clients, and also no awareness that many staff were, despite their efforts, far from competent.

As a result of changed perceptions of disabled people and their needs, it is now recognised that effective help is dependent upon worker skills. In some western countries this recognition has resulted in the rapid growth of tertiary level courses for residential workers, and an insistence that those promoted to senior positions in residential facilities have residential qualifications.

In general, however, the number of helpers with specific training in residential work remains quite small and so there is a need for the development of a variety of organisationally based forms of training.

Who needs to be trained?

The short answer to this question is every individual directly or indirectly involved in the provision of services. For those in the residential sector training should be provided for:

- boards of management
- workers in management positions
- workers with formal qualifications in disciplines not directly focused on the residential task, such as social workers, occupational therapists, psychologists, nurses and teachers
- direct care workers
- ancillary workers
- volunteers.

The level and scope of training for each group should be related to positions, responsibilities and previous training. In ideal situations, each worker should have an individual training program which is regularly reviewed and updated.

Why train workers?

The benefits of trained staff in residential situations are apprarent on four levels:

- benefits for clients: trained helpers are aware of client need and capable of providing appropriate assistance to enhance personal and social development and a positive lifestyle
- benefits for colleagues: effectively trained workers understand the relevance of teamwork and possess skills to work effectively alongside others
- benefits for organisations: trained staff have the potential to be relatively objective about what is happening within an organisation, and so can contribute to the evaluation of its effectiveness
- benefits for the individual worker: the confidence that comes with training enables individuals to be more effective. On a personal level, the trained helper has:

— skills necessary to succeed and thus to experience considerable job satisfaction
— a level of attainment which brings recognition, high personal regard and confidence

Forms of training

Among the ways in which training can be provided are through:

- continuous on the job training, for example:
  — staff meetings and seminars
  — individual supervisory sessions with managers and consultants
  — working alongside competent and trained colleagues
  — lectures, films and outside speakers
  — literature such as books, journals, training packages and specially prepared documents
- visits to other residential resources
- short periods of work experience in other settings
- conferences, short courses and workshops
- part-time and full-time tertiary studies.

Content of training programs

The content of training programs will vary considerably according to individual need. Among the areas that may be included are:

- information about the disabilities of clients assisted by the workers in question
- the place and function of residential services in overall responses to disabled people
- working with families
- programming
- the use of specific helping techniques
- creating beneficial residential contexts
- interpersonal relationships
- functioning in interdisciplinary teams
- managing staff.

Who can assist in training?

A wide range of people both within and external to residences can assist in the training of staff including:

- staff development personnel
- consultants and experts
- members of staff with expertise in specific areas
- clients and disabled people's groups
- relatives and parent groups.

HOURS OF DIRECT CARE WORKERS

The quality of client lives is dependent upon factors related to the hours of duty of direct care staff, including:

- the time at which they commence and terminate periods of duty
- the length of working shifts
- intervals between periods of duty
- length of holidays.

In the past, duty rosters were established not on the basis of client need but staff need or organisational convenience. As a result, residential life has been shaped around staff rosters and clients have suffered. Among practices that have been detrimental to clients have been:

- three rigid eight-hour shifts each day
- excessively long and exhausting periods on duty, making it impossible for helpers to effectively assist clients
- insufficient staff being available at the important and busy times of the day
- permitting workers to organise hours of duty to suit themselves
- continual shifting of staff from section to section to accommodate overall staffing needs
- allowing staff to work long periods to accumulate days off or holidays.

If staff are to assist clients effectively, their hours of duty should reflect client need. Among the more important aspects to be considered in devising and managing duty rosters are:

- general flexibility of duty hours
- availability of direct care workers at peak times such as early mornings, evenings, and

meal times; and a consequent reduction of workers on duty during the day if clients are out, and at nights if clients require little assistance
- allocation of staff to particular units and groups of clients rather than continual movement of staff for organisational convenience
- spacing of hours of duty to prevent excessively long periods at work or away from it
- adequate holidays to enable breaks to be taken at least twice yearly rather than in one large block
- establishing a holiday roster so that staff holidays are spaced throughout the year and not all taken at the one time
- establishing minimum staffing levels, and use of support and management staff in direct care worker roles to maintain them
- control of staff rosters by senior staff so that exchanges in duty hours are not made at the expense of clients
- ensuring that all staff absences are know to appropriate senior staff and unofficial absences followed up
- allocating time for meetings.

BOARDS OF MANAGEMENT

This section considers a range of issues relating to the nature and functioning of boards and committees managing residential facilities. Since there is considerable variation in the composition, function and responsibilities of boards these issues can be discussed only in general ways. All boards, however, whatever their terms of reference, should be oriented to client need and be tasked with developing policies consistent with contemporary approaches to disabled people.

Issues discussed are grouped under the following headings:

Responsibilities of boards
Membership of boards
Membership requirements
Tenure of members
Involvement in residential life.

Responsibilities of boards

Among the more significant responsibilities of boards and committees will be:

- determining and documenting formal goals of residences
- establishing day-to-day operational policies and standards of good practice
- providing finance and resources
- administering funds
- selecting heads of residences and possibly other senior workers
- advising and supporting the head of an organisation or residence
- ensuring good personnel practice
- developing community interest and involvement in a residence.

Membership of boards

It is important to ensure that membership of boards is as representative as possible and that all members have voting rights. Among those involved in residential life who should be represented by individuals of their own choosing are:

- clients
- relevant parent groups
- direct care staff.

Membership should also include interested and aware people from the community, and one or more individuals recognised as having expertise in relation to clients assisted by the organisation or residence. Members should be drawn from a broad age range, from both sexes, and from different occupational backgrounds. The only interests members should have in common will be membership of a board; they should not be associated beyond it by business, religious or professional interests.

Membership requirements

All members of boards should have the potential to make significant contributions to the life of a residence. Individuals elected or co-opted will possess the following attributes:

- have a genuine interest in and concern for the client group being assisted
- have an enlightened understanding of their needs
- be willing to become an involved and contributing member of a board
- be able to effectively represent a residence.

Tenure of members

A time limit should be placed on individual membership to enable the recruitment of people with new and significant contributions to make and phasing out of those with little to offer. This can be achieved and continuity maintained where a percentage of positions becomes vacant each year.

Involvement in residential life

In addition to formal responsibilities described above, outside members of boards should become involved in the life of a residence so as to get to know clients. Where this has not happened before, it can be initiated by having an occasional formal meal to which one or two board members are invited. This will provide them with an opportunity to establish a base for more informal future involvement.

22

Dimensions of accountability

There was until recently no expectation that organisations assisting disabled people should be accountable for the services they provided. Because their existence was interpreted as a manifestation of a humane and caring society it was taken for granted that whatever happened within them was of benefit to clients. As a result, residential facilities were left to operate entirely as they saw fit and only ever questioned when extreme forms of abuse came to light.

Major changes in approaches to disabled people have today created a critical climate in relation to existing services, and particularly those provided in the residential context. This is reflected in:

- a willingness of governments to initiate enquiries into the operation of residential facilities, to be judgemental of them and to publish their findings
- the interest the media takes in residential care and its exposure of what it sees as abuse and poor quality services
- action by clients, parents, relatives and pressure groups to achieve better services
- demands by helpers employed in or associated with residential contexts that services be improved
- the setting of standards for accreditation or licencing
- the use of legal processes to challenge service deficiences

213

- a general and increasing expectation that organisations providing services should be accountable for what they do.

This chapter is concerned with the final point and explores three ways in which accountability can be pursued.

THE IDEA OF ACCOUNTABILITY

The notion of accountability asserts that those providing services should be answerable for what they do, that is, they have no right to provide only that which they see fit but should subject themselves and what they do to the scrutiny of others.

In seeking to become more accountable, residential services should be sensitive to the views of a number of groups including:

- clients, parents, relatives and advocates
- those employed in helping services, including residential staff
- organisations funding services and resources
- the wider society through the media and legal services.

There are a number of ways of increasing the accountability of residential services. The three approaches discussed in this chapter are those which can be introduced and developed through management initiatives. They are:

> *Contracting*
> *Advocacy*
> *Complaints.*

CONTRACTING

The introduction of contracting to human services is a recent development. In the context of assisting disabled people a contract can be defined as:

> *a verbal or written agreement or understanding between two or more parties concerning the provision of specific forms of assistance.*

While contracts in the business world have formal and legal components, these dimensions are not appropriate in service provision. Contracts are not meant to compel disabled people and those assisting them to do certain things but rather to achieve:

- helpful discussion of need and the ways in which it can be met
- the commitment of clients, families and helpers to the provision of specific forms of help
- an understanding that individuals should be accountable for what they do.

Where contracts are not being met by one or more of the parties involved, it is, for the most part, unhelpful to respond in a judgemental or negative way. It is better to explore reasons for failure and perhaps acknowledge that the original contract may have been unrealistic and unattainable. This will lead to discussion and renegotiation of the contract which should make it more helpful.

Contracts relating to services provided by residential facilities should be negotiated and freely entered into. Some notions of contracting view contracts as a way of obtaining client compliance. Not only is this contrary to the basic principles of contracting, it is inconsistent with contemporary approaches and thus a blatant form of manipulation.

Contracts can be made between a wide range of individuals and groups involved in residential contexts, for example:

> *Between clients and helpers.* These contracts may concern:

- provision by helpers of appropriate assistance as detailed in individual plans
- clients working on areas detailed in individual plans
- clients accepting greater responsibility for aspects of daily life.

> *Between families and helpers.* These contracts may concern:

- agreement about reasons for residential assistance and grounds for concluding placement

- contacts to be maintained and assistance provided by families
- services to be provided to families by helpers
- accommodation to be found on conclusion of placement.

Among clients. These contracts may concern:

- common and acceptable standards of behaviour
- individual and group responsibilities for aspects of daily life.

Between managers and direct care workers. These contracts may concern:

- provision of support by managers
- working together to improve relationships
- direct care staff undertaking to meet needs of clients as detailed in individual plans.

Among direct care workers. These contracts may concern:

- supporting one another
- completing tasks when on duty
- attending meetings
- sharing information.

Perhaps the value of contracting comes not from the actual formation of a contract but from discussions preceding it. Where, for example, clients, appropriate close relatives and helpers meet to identify what help is needed and the kinds of contracts that may be appropriate, a whole new way of relating develops.

ADVOCACY

Discussions on advocacy and the advocate role appear in a number of chapters in this book. What is written here is a more general consideration of advocacy as it relates to the concept of accountability.

Like contracting, advocacy in human services has a short history, with most developments having taken place in North America. Before considering its relevance to services for disabled people, it is necessary to have some understanding of what it means.

The terms advocate and advocacy are related to notions of justice. People appearing before criminal or civil courts, and lacking sufficient expertise to plead their own case, engage others to represent them, to be, in other words, their advocates. The task of advocates is to see the alleged issue or offence not from all sides but from the client's perspective, and to seek to persuade others to see it that way also. Thus, in practice, opposing parties are represented in court proceedings by biased advocates who dispute in the interests of those they represent. Their task and the process in which they take part are understood and recognised by all involved and seen as essential in the attainment of justice.

When this concept is applied to services for disabled people, advocates become individuals with responsibility for representing clients. They are expected to view services provided for clients from the client's point of view, and to take action wherever they believe deficiencies to exist.

In practical terms, advocates represent the interests of clients by:

- being aware of client rights and seeking to uphold them
- becoming informed about the lives of clients and services provided
- participating in meetings where the needs or interests of clients are being considered
- accompanying or representing clients at individual planning meetings
- taking action on the complaints of clients
- teaching clients to relate on an equal basis to helpers and to act successfully on their own behalf.

The necessity for advocacy in relation to residential services reflects not only dissatisfaction with past practices but also an awareness that organisational constraints often make it difficult for helpers to give priority to the needs of clients. Thus it may be only as a result of the activities of advocates that client need can be placed first.

The awareness of the counter-productive nature of organisational life has resulted in the introduction of citizen advocacy. This involves the recruitment of concerned and enlightened members of the community to act as advocates on behalf of individual clients. After getting to know clients and the residences in which they live citizen advocates, where necessary, bring pressure to bear on organisations and helpers to ensure clients receive the best possible assistance. Recruiting and training citizen advocates is seen as a responsibility of organisations providing residential services. This reflects an awareness that:

- external pressure is often necessary, even where helpers believe they are effectively helping clients, to ensure that essential services are provided
- recognising the needs of clients may sometimes be dependent upon the perceptions of those not directly involved in the helping process
- all levels of staff should be open and receptive to criticism and complaint
- advocates will act in ways that sometimes create difficulties for helpers.

There is a second and quite different way in which the notion of advocacy can be used to the benefit of disabled people living in residential settings. Helpers can be encouraged to view their role as including an advocate dimension, and this is an issue that is discussed in Chapter 17. While taking on an advocate role will at times involve workers in a conflict of interest between the requirements of employers and the needs of the clients, if should not, for this reason, be seen as inappropriate. If worker advocacy is to become a reality it will necessitate certain changes in the way organisations operate, in the way helpers view their task, undertake their work and relate to one another and in the way managers relate to and deal with workers.

COMPLAINTS

Most organisations experience considerable difficulty in dealing with complaints. Criticisms implied by them and the problems they cause seem to make matters worse rather than better. While it may seem somewhat paradoxical, organisations providing services for disabled people should respond positively to complaints since they provide information which can lead to the improvement of services.

There is a need for helping organisations to devise effective ways of responding to complaints. The manner in which they do so is likely to differ considerably from past practices where complaints were, more often than not, neutralised by:

- viewing the person making the complaint as malevolent and a trouble maker. Thus the complainant became the problem and not the issue being complained about
- exposing or dealing with complainants in ways that were detrimental to them
- allowing those about whom complaints were made to deal with them
- scapegoating workers at the bottom of an organisation by placing all blame on them
- suppressing a complaint or denying its truth as an act of loyalty to others or to protect oneself.

Failure to respond effectively to complaints only serves to sustain poor quality services. While complaints may create difficulties, they should be responded to in a professional way whatever they are about, however they have been made and irrespective of the status of those making them.

Complaints are made by many people such as clients, relatives, those representing clients, helpers, members of the public and the media. Those making complaints should be seen as having a right to do so, be guaranteed confidentiality and in no way victimised for their actions. Concern for the personal consequences of making a complaint often leads to anonymity or a refusal to commit a complaint to writing; neither situation should be sufficient justification for inaction.

Dealing with complaints

There are two ways of responding to complaints: informally and formally. The response chosen will be dependent upon the seriousness of the complaint and also, to some extent, the wishes of the person making it.

Informal responses

Where a complaint is seen as relatively minor, it can be dealt with informally by the worker to whom it has been made. If that worker is unable to deal with it, the complaint should be passed to the appropriate senior person. Often where complaints are minor, little action is necessary beyond acknowledging the complaint to have been justified, and taking action to ensure that the circumstances giving rise to it do not recur. Responding effectively to minor complaints not only brings about ongoing improvements in services, it makes helpers more conscious of the assistance they are providing and so contributes to a general improvement in services.

Formal responses

Complaints of a more serious kind should be responded to according to a formally established procedure. Such a procedure will be drawn up by organisations responsible for residential services and made public. An appropriate procedure will detail:

- action by the person to whom the complaint was made
- the manner in which complaints should be investigated. An investigation should be carried out by two or three people with no involvement in or responsibility for the workers or the residence in question
- action by those undertaking the investigation. The following stages should feature in most investigations:

Stage one: the individual making the complaint will be interviewed to obtain full details of it

Stage two: All people involved will be interviewed and asked to give their account of the situation and events relating to it. Each person should know the purpose of the interview beforehand and have someone present of their own choosing to act as witness or to represent them. This person can be a colleague, a union employee or, where a serious complaint has been made, a solicitor. If a worker is likely to make an incriminating statement, an interview should not proceed without adequate representation

Stage three: A report of the investigation will be presented to the appropriate senior manager. It will detail grounds for the complaint, the stages of the enquiry, findings, include copies of statements and conclude with a summary and recommendations

- action by the manager receiving the report. Action should be taken in whatever way is considered appropriate. Whatever the course of action:
  — the person making the complaint should be informed of its outcome. If he/she remains dissatisfied, information should be provided about further steps that can be taken
  — those about whom the complaint was made should be informed of the outcome of the investigation and action to be taken. They should be left in no doubt as to whether they personally are or are not being held responsible.

PART | FIVE

Glossary

The terms in this glossary include not only those appearing in preceding chapters but also many others frequently used in work with disabled people. It is impossible to include all such terms and no attempt has been made to do so. Those selected are those which are used in a precise or unusual way, provide additional information or which reflect contemporary thinking about the ways in which disabled people can be assisted. Discussion of each term has been kept brief, and where a term has been considerd in detail in the book, that discussion has not been repeated. The numbers in brackets following a term denote the chapter where discussion of it can be found.

Abnormal   A term used about individuals who are perceived to differ in some way from others, to the extent of being considered qualitatively different. A wide range of factors have been used to define people as abnormal, the more usual being personal impairment and exceptional behaviour. Disabled people have been viewed as abnormal because of their disability and behaviour attributed to it.

While many definitions of abnormality are claimed to be based on objective criteria, all definitions have the function of denoting difference, inferiority and unacceptability. Each is derived from beliefs about individual wholeness and acceptability, and while some may appear common to a society, that in no way negates their judgemental function.

Since all conceptions of abnormality are socially based, it is likely to be the case that when wider belief systems change so will these conceptions. Considerable change has, in fact, taken place in western societies over the past twenty years, and beliefs about many groups traditionally seen as abnormal, particularly disabled people, are now quite different. Today disabled people are increasingly recognised as having an entitlement to live and function as do others, thereby implying a rejection of orientations that suggest abnormality.

See also Deviants, Mainstream society, Normalisation, Normality

Access   In the past disabled people were rejected from society because they were considered incapable of contributing to it. This led to the erection of considerable psychological, social and physical barriers to reinforce their exclusion, many of which still exist and continue to handicap them. Now that disabled people are seen as having a right to participate fully in society it is necessary to remove these barriers.

The term access denotes this right to be included in mainstream education, work, housing, leisure and medical services. For physically disabled people with mobility problems, it also denotes the need to provide appropriate assistance and to modify buildings to make physical access possible.

See also Disability, Handicap, Least restrictive alternative, Mainstreaming, Normalisation

Accountability (Ch. 22)   Over the past twenty years the operation of many organisations assisting disabled people has been closely examined by academic research, and by government enquiries and court actions. This examination has frequently revealed poor quality services and dehumanising patterns of residential life. One explanation as to why this should have been so has been based on the recognition that those providing services have never had to account for their actions, but have been free to operate entirely as they saw fit. Over a period of many years, and probably several generations of workers, this resulted in a degree of insensitivity that rendered workers incapable of recognising what they were really doing to disabled people. For this reason, it is now asserted that all organisations providing services should become accountable, or answerable, for what they do.

See also Advocacy Complaints systems, Contract.

Activity therapy centre   *See* Adult training centre

Adaptive behaviour   The ability to meet the standards of the wider society. Functioning in mainstream society involves participating in situations where there is an expectation, and often an obligation, to behave in new or different ways.

Such expectations and obligations are usually associated with behaviour appropriate to age, social roles and cultural contexts. The extent to which individuals are able to meet these standards influences their participation in social life.

Many disabled people have difficulties in adaptive behaviour because of limitations that are a consequence of disability and the handicapping nature of society. For these reasons the notion of adaptive behaviour can be a useful way of identifying such limitations and the kinds of assistance needed to overcome them.

See also Independence, Role

Admission process (Ch. 4)   In the past, most children and adults entering residential accommodation were subjected to dehumanising admission processes (Goffman, 1961). Often this involved being bathed, having hair cropped, removal of personal, possessions, being dressed in institutional clothing and formalised documentation of personal details. The impact of such a process on the individual was usually quite devastating, and symbolically it represented conversion from the person he/she was before admission to a cleansed, uniformly presented and compliant inmate.

While such rituals are now rare, many residences continue to find it necessary to set in motion a formalised process the day a client moves into a residence. It is important to ensure that whatever the process, it is humane and personalised.

See also Dehumanising, Institutionalisation, Ritual.

Adoption   Providing young children, unable to be raised for the remainder of their childhood by their natural parents, with permanent substitute parents. Adoption is a legal process, and once a child has been adopted the adopting parents have the same legal rights and responsibilities for the child as do natural parents.

Contemporary beliefs about the needs of disabled children assert that adoption should be considered essential for younger children permanently separated from their natural parents, even to the point of permitting it against the wishes of natural parents. This approach is based on the belief that a child can develop successfully only within the context and as a full member of a family. It is argued that no matter how good an alternative may be, whether it be foster or residential care, there can be no adequate substitute for a childhood spent in a wholesome and secure family environment.

See also Foster care, Short-term care

Adult training centre   A day centre for disabled people providing a range of activities to enhance personal and social development. The programs of adult training centres include vocational, educational, recreational and social experiences. Increasing emphasis is being placed on the need for flexible programs that are client centred, and the elimination of activities, such as repetitive and boring contract work, that have no relevance or value to clients.

See also Client-centred approach, Day care services, Sheltered workshop.

Advocacy (Chs 17 & 22)   Acting with and on behalf of disabled people to ensure that their individual rights, needs and interests are met.

The introduction of advocacy is a consequence of:
- past denial of the rights of disabled people
- the failure of organisations to recognise and respond to disabled people as individuals
- an awareness that organisational factors often make it impossible for helpers to take a client-centred approach.

The application of the notion of advocacy to human services has been modelled on its use in the legal context where an advocate is expected to see issues from the point of view of the client and, wherever possible, without any conflict of interests.

There are several ways in which advocacy is being developed:
- citizen advocacy — using enlightened and capable members of society, with no responsibilities in the settings in which clients are assisted, to represent clients
- agency advocacy — influencing organisations to the point where they view their major objective as meeting the needs clients identify for themselves
- helper advocacy — recognising that an essential dimension of the helper role is to represent the interests of clients to the point of actively seeking an improvement in the quality of assistance provided by the organisations of which they are members
- client advocacy — not advocacy in the strict sense of the term, but an idea that remains useful in that it identifies the need to develop the abilities of clients so that they are able to act on their own behalf in dealings with helping organisations.

See also Client-centred approach

Alienation   A sense of powerlessness, isolation, meaninglessness and self-estrangement that is caused by living in a society or being a member of a group or organisation that is constantly changing to the point where an individual cannot identify with or feel part of it.

Allocation team (Ch. 4)   A group responsible for the allocation of specific services. Growth in the use of allocation teams reflects an awareness that services should be made available only to clients whose need for them has been demonstrated, and in some order of priority where demand exceeds availability. Membership of allocation teams includes a permanent group of helpers who are able to contribute meaningfully to discussions about client need, and additional members when particular clients are being considered. Included in the latter group will be clients, their close relatives and advocates, particularly when residential provision is being considered.

See also Intake system, Priority systems

Assessment (Ch. 6)   A process that involves the collection, organisation and interpretation of information about clients in order to identify needs and ways in which they can be met. Assessment in the residential context is no longer viewed as a predetermined and comprehensive process to be applied to all clients on admission, but as something that should be individualised and ongoing. It therefore follows that if a specific form of assessment is to be used with a client it must be of relevance to that client's life situation. Assessment processes that simply categorise, or which provide information that has little relevance for clients, are of little value.

See also Category, Checklist, Individual plan

Asylum   In its original meaning, an asylum was a place or sanctuary, refuge or shelter from society. Nineteenth century institutions into which disabled people were placed were called asylums because of the generally accepted belief that such people needed to be separated from society for their own good. This argument served, in fact, to justify the permanent removal of many disabled people from society and their retention in custodial institutions. This term is now seen as an inappropriate description of any form of residential accommodation.

Attendant care   Personal assistance provided to a severely disabled person living in the community. The assistant is a paid employee, hired by the disabled person to help with aspects of daily life such as bathing, dressing, toileting, shopping, meal preparation and domestic chores. That nature of the assistance is determined by the disabled person, not by the assistant or by helping agencies.

Attention span   The length of time an individual is able to concentrate on a particular activity or task. While attention span varies considerably according to age, task and degree of motivation, many intellectually disabled people, because of their disabilities or past experiences, do have shorter attention spans than others. This fact needs to be taken into account when helping them to develop new skills.

See also Programming

Authoritarian   This term is used about individuals who hold rigid sets of beliefs about life, personal responsibilities and interpersonal relationships and who seek to impose them upon others. The beliefs of authoritarian people are usually conservative, supportive of relationships based on traditional notions of authority, focused on perserving what they believe to be good and hostile to ideas contrary to their own. While there are many problems over the definition of this term, it is nevertheless useful in that it provides a way of understanding the beliefs and behaviour of individuals, and particularly those holding management positions in organisations who operate in controlling and directive ways whatever the issues, context or workers involved.

See also Directive management, Non-authoritarian, Participative management

Autism   A developmental condition which is characterised by severe difficulties in relationships and adaptive behaviour. An autistic person will manifest many of the following behaviours to a degree that is considered not typical: poor communication, limited attention span, avoidance of physical and eye contact, inappropriate social behaviour. The term autism has never been defined in any satisfactory way and should be used with caution.

Behaviour modification (Ch. 8)   A form of instruction, normally undertaken in the context of structured programming, which systematically uses reward and punishment to promote learning. In the past fifteen years behaviour modification has been used extensively with disabled children and adults who, because of limitations resulting from disability or earlier experiences, have been unable to learn in the more usual and natural ways.

It is important to ensure that whatever forms of reward are used in behaviour modification programs are those which are not the basic necessities of life, and that any punishments are neither excessive nor abnormal. While punishment may have an occasional part to play in assisting clients to learn, it is more desirable and more effective to concentrate on rewarding appropriate behaviour than punishing inappropriate behaviour.

See also Programming, Punishment, Reinforcement

Beneficial environment (Ch. 10)   A normalised living environment that has been consciously created and maintained in order to meet the needs of clients and provide a decent pattern of life. The idea of a beneficial environment is of significance in the provision of residential services as it draws attention to the importance of the setting in which disabled people live, their relationships with others and their pattern of daily life.

Blaming the victim   A phrase describing the way in which certain individuals tend to be blamed and punished for personal conditions, lifestyles or behaviour for which they are not, in fact, directly responsible (Ryan, 1976). In other words, many of the problems and difficulties associated with individuals defined as deviant are a consequence of factors entirely beyond their control. In the ways they are dealt with, however, this fact is usually denied and they are treated as if they were to blame. An example of victim blaming is the belief that unemployed people are to be blamed for their situation despite the fact that work is unavailable for most of them. When applied to disabled people this idea reveals attitudes underlying past approaches, that is, as if they had brought their disabilities upon themselves, and it also explains why past approaches were often more punitive than helpful.

See also Deviants

Boards of management (Ch. 21)   Groups of people with overall managerial responsibility for the ways in whch organisations provide assistance to disabled people. Boards of management, committees or councils usually comprise both elected and co-opted members. Two major criticisms of many boards today are that some members have little awareness of the needs of the client groups their organisations are assisting, and that membership is unrepresentative.

Case manager (Ch. 5)   A helper in an organisation or residence who has responsibility for ensuring that individual client plans are prepared, implemented and reviewed.

See also Individual plan, Key worker

Category   In the past disabled people were understood and responded to according to categories, that is, distinct groups delineated by what were identified as their major defects. Physically disabled people were usually identified in terms of medical conditions such as cerebral palsy or spina bifida, whereas intellectually disabled people were categorised according to assessed intelligence, resulting in placement of one of four categories; mild, moderate, severe and profound retardation. It was assumed without question that all those included in a particular category had identical needs. Objections to the use of categories are based on the fact that they emanate from and reinforce static conceptions of disabled people and thus are self-fulfilling prophesies. For these reasons they are, wherever possible, best avoided as a basis for service provision.

See also Classification, Intellectual disability, Intelligence tests, Labelling, Self-fulfilling prophesy, Stereotype.

Centrally-based services (Ch. 3)   Provision of services and resources in large towns and cities. Contemporary approaches emphasise the need to move from centrally-based to regionally-based services to enable disabled people to be assisted while living at home or in their usual neighbourhoods.

See also Community care, Community-based services, Regionally-based services

Cerebral palsy   A group of conditions caused by damage to the central nervous system before, during or following birth. Cerebral palsy impairs motor functioning, with the person affected likely to have one or more of the following problems: tight muscles, poor co-ordination, jerking uncontrollable movements or poor balance. The resultant disability can range from mild to severe, and may be accompanied by other disabilities such as poor perception, difficulties with verbal communication or intellectual disability.

Chaining (Ch. 7)   A method of teaching the sequential steps of a complex task. To enable a client to learn a complete task it may be necessary to break the task into a number of skill stages. The task can then be taught in one of three ways:
- from first to last stage — forward chaining
- from last to first stage — backward chaining
- from simple to complex stages — developmental chaining.

See also Task analysis

Charities   Organisations assisting disabled people who rely on public donations for all or part of their income. While charities feature prominently in work with disabled people, it is important to recognise that they sometimes fail to meet need because:
- provision of services has often been related more to moral judgements about clients than actual need
- a major function of charities has been to benefit those who contribute by enabling them to feel that the act of giving exempts them from further involvement and commitment
- many helpers have expected 'aren't they wonderful' type responses from society and gratitude from clients
- clients can be trapped by conceptions of themselves that are an outcome of charity, that is, not as having needs that should be met as a matter of right but as being dependent upon the goodwill of others for assistance. This reinforces feelings of less eligibility within society, among disabled people themselves and those assisting them.

While charities will continue to play a significan part in the provision of services, if their contributions are to be consistent with contemporary approaches they should seek to:
- meet need wherever it may be found, and not be bound by the values, beliefs and morals of those who donate to or who manage them
- co-operate rather than compete with other organisations providing services in their localities

- ensure that need exists for the services they wish to make available.

See also Comprehensive planning

Checklist (Ch. 6)   A list of adaptive behaviours or skills considered appropriate for socially competent people against which the capabilities of disabled people can be compared. Checklists are a form of assessment and are useful in contributing to a clearer understanding of what clients are able to do. Before using checklists they should be discussed with clients and client approval sought. Findings should be interpreted with caution and should never serve to justify the imposition of behaviour change programmes.

See also Assessment, Programming

Classification   This term is very similar in meaning to category. When used as a verb, that is, the act of classifying disabled people, it refers to the means by which they are assigned to categories. In the past considerable effort went into devising classification procedures, the most popular and widely used being medical diagnosis and intelligence testing. Classifying disabled people and responding to them in terms of categories is no longer favoured because it results in stereotyping and denial of individual need.

See also Category, Intelligence tests, Labelling, Self-fulfilling prophesy, Stereotype

Client   A client is a person in need of or receiving assistance from any form of helping agency. While this is by no means an ideal term to use about disabled people and those close to them, it probably is an improvement on terms used in the past. Furthermore, if it is understood in the way it is used by the legal profession, that is, a client as someone who engages a competent person to act on his/her behalf, it is of considerable value in that it suggests the nature of the relationship that ought to exist between disabled people and those assisting them. From another perspective, a client is a consumer of services and therefore has consumer rights.

Client-centred approach   Structuring the operation of an organisation or residence around the needs of individual clients.

See also Organisation-centred approach, Staff-centred approach, Tradition-centred approach.

Client records (Ch. 9)   The collection and retention of information about clients and their families. All organisations and residences will probably need to keep some form of client records which will, unless strong reasons exist to the contrary, be freely available to clients, their close relatives and those representing them.

Cognitive   A term that refers to the mental processes of perceiving, thinking, remembering, reasoning, imagining and judging. Many intellectually disabled people are limited in cognitive functioning.

Community-based services   Services made available to disabled people and others assisting them while they are living in their own homes or in residences in mainstream society. Most services, apart from those provided in large, isolated residences, are seen as community-based services, and contemporary approaches stress the need for an increase in their provision.

See also Centrally-based services, Community care

Community care   A term describing the provision and use of services at the local, neighbourhood or community level. Although the notion of community care dominates most helping responses today, it is important to recognise that it is a highly problematic concept in that not only is it difficult to define, it also tends to be used in an idealistic and sentimentalised way, and from an unquestioned assumption about its desirability. As a result, both policy makers and professionals have failed to consider what community care means in practice. Of particular importance is the issue of whether community care means care *by* members of the community, or the provision of services to enable disabled people to live successfully *within* the community. The outcome of this lack of clarity in thinking has been the hasty closure of large institutions and transfer of clients to supposedly community-based facilities, regardless of whether support services are available. It has also resulted in greater emphasis on the family as the major provider for disabled people. Where disabled people have been forced to remain with or have been returned to their families without adequate support services, it has resulted in intolerable stress for families, particularly the woman in the family. Community care is, in fact, about enabling disabled people to live successfully within society and so it is dependent upon the provision of all necessary support services.
   See also Community-based services

Community integration (Ch. 13)   Participating in the everyday aspects of life and being recognised as a normal member of society. Community integration, which is integral to the concept of normalisation, is seen as a right, and essential for appropriate development. Making integration a reality necessitates helpers working to involve disabled children and adults in mainstream social life, particularly in the areas of education, work, leisure and health.
   See also Mainstreaming, Normalisation

Community residences (Ch. 11)   A general term describing accommodation for disabled people located in residential districts, and in housing typical for the neighbourhood. Community residences are seen as preferable to the more traditional forms of residential accommodation which, while sometimes located in residential districts, are architecturally so different from homes nearby that they make integration impossible.
   See also Community integration, Small community residences

Complaints systems (Ch. 22)   Formally established procedures that should be followed whenever complaints are made about any aspect of the operation of an organisation or residence assisting disabled people.

Comprehensive planning (Ch. 3)   An approach to the provision of services that begins by identifying the needs of all disabled people within an identified district or region, and which uses this information as a basis for determining the kinds of services to be provided.

Congenital   A medical term usually used to describe a disability existing before or at the time of birth. A congenital condition may or may not be hereditary.

Congregate care   A form of residential provision where large groups of disabled people are processed by staff through a tightly scheduled daily routine without choice, and without variation according to individual difference or need. While this form of provision may have appeared appropriate in the past, it is today seen as dehumanising, and considerable efforts are being made to eliminate it.
   See also Dehumanising, Institutionalisation, Total institution

Consensus decision-making   A consensus decision is one that is made by a group, and supported and implemented by each member even though some may have personal objections to or reservations about it. Consensus decision-making usually takes place in the context of teamwork where individuals are willing to modify the positions they take on issues to enable binding decisions to be made.

Consultants (Ch. 20)   Individuals, not normally employed by an organisation or residence, who are engaged to assist in clarifying what is happening, in solving problems and in contributing to the development of better services. Consultants are seen as having a significant part to play when major changes to residential services are sought. Not only have they appropriate expertise, but also, in not being members of the organisations in question, they are able to attain greater insight and act somewhat more objectively than can managers and other staff.

Contract (Ch. 22)   A verbally or formally documented understanding or agreement between two or more people concerning the provision of services to disabled people and the responsibilities of those involved.
   See also Accountability

Continuum   A way of conceptualising or explaining a range of skills, qualities, attributes, etc., in terms of degree along a scale as opposed to discrete categories. Instead of arguing, for example, that disabled people have conditions that make them dependent and which therefore prevent them ever becoming independent, a continuum enables degrees of dependence and independence to be identified.

Coping mechanisms   The ways in which individuals tend to respond to and deal with stressful events. Coping mechanisms range from those that are necessary and appropriate for the individual to those that are bizarre and destructive.

Corporal punishment (Ch. 16)   Inflicting physical pain by smacking, punching, kicking, squeezing or shaking.

Counselling   A form of help that uses discussion between clients and helpers to enable clients to better understand themselves, those close to them, their life situation and the meanings they attach to events and behaviour. The aims of the counselling process are to assist the client in attaining a helpful perspective of his/her world, to identify what specific forms of help may be needed and how that help can be obtained.

Crisis   The occurrence of certain unanticipated events in a context where one or more disabled people live or function, with which neither the disabled people themselves nor others closely associated with them can deal, and which necessitates immediate assistance from one or more helping agencies.
   See also Emergency residential care

Day care services   Forms of assistance involving attendance at a resource or centre on a day basis ranging from a few hours to seven days a week. Day care services include nurseries, kindergartens, adult training centres, activity therapy centres, sheltered workshops and social and drop-in centres. Assistance provided by such centres may take the form of child minding, nurturing, recreation, education, socialisation, skill training, work and health care.

See also Adult training centre, Sheltered workshop

Decarceration   *See* Deinstitutionalisation

Degenerative   Decline in physical or intellectual functioning as a result of a specific condition.

Dehumanising   A living situation can be described as dehumanising when it deprives one or more people of a pattern of life essential for meeting basic needs. Failure to provide adequate or appropriate shelter, food, warmth, clothing, personal relationships, intimacy, individualisation, dignity or privacy justifies a situation being described as dehumanising.

See also Depersonalising lifestyle, Individualisation, Intimacy, Privacy

Deinstitutionalisation   A term describing the policy of closing large congregate residential facilities and returning disabled people to their families or moving them to community-based accommodation.

See also Community care, Institutionalisation, Community residences

Democratic living (Ch. 10)   Involving disabled people in decisions about daily life in the residences in which they live. Democratic living is considered to be essential in that it is consistent with the basic right of adults to control their lives and it enables disabled people to develop the capacity to exercise responsibility and act in mature ways.

Demonstration (Ch. 8)   A form of instruction where tasks or skills are demonstrated to clients in ways that enable them to comprehend what is involved so that they can successfully imitate what they have observed. Showing disabled people how to do things is part of daily living and also features in programming.

See also Modelling, Programming

Depersonalising lifestyle   The imposition of a pattern of life on disabled people which denies individuality, choice and opportunity to develop a sense of dignity and self-worth.

See also Congregate care, Dehumanising, Institutionalisation, Self-concept

Deprivation   Taking away from people the basic comforts and significant dimensions of life. Many clients have been deprived as a result of moving from home to institutional care. This term is often confused with privation. The latter term more accurately describes the experiences of disabled people who have never enjoyed the basic comforts of life, as has been the case for those who have lived virtually the whole of their lives in congregate residences.

See also Congregate care, Dehumanising, Depersonalised lifestyle, Institutionalisation, Privation

Developmental approach (Ch. 2)   The developmental approach views disabled people as being no different from other members of society in having a capacity for growth, development and maturation. This notion is seen

as a key idea on which approaches to disabled people should be based, and stands as a rejection of traditional approaches based on beliefs implying an inability to develop beyond a child-like level. It also implies that disabled adults should be dealt with in an age-appropriate way and only involved in activities that reflect their adult status.

See also Maturity

Developmental disability   A disability that is congenital or which develops in the formative years and may be permanent.

See also Congenital

Developmental stages   An analysis of the way in which people develop suggests a series of stages in physical, intellectual, social and emotional development. When the development of disabled people is explored in relation to these stages a useful indication can be gained of the extent to which they may be impaired and so require specialised assistance.

Deviants   Individuals who are unable to or who choose not to meet the standards their society sets for acceptability, and against whom some negative action is taken. Among groups traditionally defined as deviant have been those with emotional difficulties, young offenders, aged and physically and intellectually disabled people. It is asserted today that these groups should no longer be viewed as deviants worthy of negative treatment but as disadvantaged people in need of assistance.

See also Abnormal, Blaming the victim

Diagnosis   The process by which a disease or illness is identified. Because of the dominance of medically trained workers in the care of disabled people, it was taken for granted that before treatment or therapy could be administered, a client's condition required accurate diagnosis. This led to a preoccupation with ways of identifying and categorising disabilities and to quite static conceptions of disabled people. While it remains necessary to identify need before providing assistance, the processes involved are quite different from medical or clinical diagnosis.

See also Category, Classification, Medicalisation, Therapy, Treatment

Dignity of risk (Ch. 10)   The belief that since disabled people are essentially no different from other members of society, they are entitled to experience situations and encounter aspects of life that may be a potential or actual threat to their well-being. This is not to assert that they should be placed in dangerous situations, but that a normal and essential aspect of life, and one which is crucial to appropriate development, is the risk dimension. This belief stands in opposition to past practices where disabled people were over-protected and denied any dimension of risk in their lives.

See also Normalisation, Least restrictive alternative

Direct care workers   Workers in residential settings who spend the greater part of their time working directly with disabled people. The use of the word 'care' in this title is sometimes seen as implying that direct care workers exist to do things to or for disabled people. While this is not intended, the lack of clarity does highlight the difficulty in finding terms that are consistent with the beliefs on which contemporary approaches to disabled people are based.

Directive management (Ch. 18)   An approach to the management of workers and the resolution of organisational issues based on the belief that a person in a senior position has a right, indeed an obligation, to instruct subordinates as to how they should undertake their work. Directive managers take for granted that the power and authority invested in them is theirs to exercise and that junior workers are being obstructive when they fail to do as they are told.
See also Authoritarian, Participative management

Disability   A functional restriction caused by some form of impairment, for example, an inability to walk due to spinal unjury.
See also Handicap, Impairment

Discrimination   This term, from the point of view of its dictionary definition, is a neutral one. It means the act of distinguishing or differentiating between objects or people. In relation to its application to people in the context of social life it is usually used in the sense of *discriminating against*, that is, denying an individual or group equal treatment, opportunity or reward because of some perceived incompetence, defect or inferiority. Disabled people have clearly been discriminated against in the past, and it is now asserted that their rights can be realised only by discriminating in favour of them, that is, through *positive discrimination*.
See also Positive discrimination

Disturbed   A term frequently used about people who behave in strange, abnormal or unacceptable ways. It is a label that tends to be applied, not just to the behaviour in question, but also about the person in total, thus locating him/her in a deviant and abnormal status. Few if any people are disturbed to the extent implied by the conventional use of this label and to continue to describe them as disturbed is to be unhelpful to them. It is more appropriate to think in terms of disturbed behaviour or disturbing experiences.
See also Deviants, Labelling, Stereotype

Down's syndrome   A congenital condition caused by an abnormal chromosome pattern. This results in clearly identifiable physical features such as slanted eyes placed far apart, slightly smaller head than is usual, short arms and legs in comparison with the rest of the body and a large tongue. The Down's syndrome person usually looks older than he/she is and often experiences heart or respiratory problems. Down's syndrome usually affects intellectual functioning in some way, but the range in impairment is very considerable. Some people are able to function quite normally whereas others are so impaired as to be rendered profoundly disabled.

Early intervention   Provision of special assistance to infants and pre-school children, and often to their families, where the children or families are disadvantaged in some way. Early intervention is based on the knowledge that if such assistance is given effectively it can reduce the longer-term consequences of disadvantage. Early intervention programs are crucial for most disabled children.

Emergency residential care (Ch. 4)   Provision of residential accommodation on an immediate and unplanned basis to assist a disabled person, or to relieve a family or group with whom the person lives, because of the development of an unforseen situation making it impossible for the person to receive adequate care by remaining where he/she is.
See also Crisis, Respite care

Emotional manipulation   Controlling others through the manipulation of feelings or emotions. This can be attained, for example, by creating feelings of guilt and by exclusion from normal social interactions. The anxiety resulting from such treatment usually induces those manipulated to behave in the desired ways. While emotional manipulation probably features in all relationships and socialisation experiences, clear limits should be set on the extent to which it is used by workers as a means of controlling clients.

Environmental deprivation   Inadequate ştimulation of a child or adult in their everyday environment to the extent of having detrimental consequences for their development, functioning and self-concept. Many of the larger congregate residences of the past were environmentally depriving.
See also Congregate care, Deprivation, Institution, Institutionalisation, Self-concept

Epilepsy   A condition affecting the central nervous system which manifests itself by fits. In their more extreme forms, fits result in convulsions and loss of consciousness. Epilepsy can usually be controlled by medication.

Eugenics (Ch. 1)   A field of study which is interested in the inherited characteristics of the human being and its relevance to the development of the human race. The ideas of the eugenicists were popular in the early part of the twentieth century and contributed to social policies reinforcing inferior treatment of many minority groups, particularly disabled people.

Evolution   A theory asserting that all forms of life survive only when they are able to adapt successfully to continually changing environmental factors that threaten them. Among such threatening factors are changes in food supply, climate and predators. Since life is in a constant state of change the process of continuous adaptation leads, over a period of time, to the development of more advanced forms of life.
   In the nineteenth century the theory of evolution was applied to society suggesting that it, too, was in a constant state of change, and that the industrialised form of society was more advanced than the pre-industrial one. One major function of this argument was to justify changes in society caused by industrialisation and to negate its harmful consequences. According to those supporting the idea of an evolving society, individuals who could not compete successfully and provide for themselves were the unfit who, by the natural order of things, were not meant to survive. This theory, not surprisingly, was applied to disabled people reinforcing hostile attitudes towards and negative treatment of them.
See also Industrialisation

Extrinsic reinforcement   *See* Reinforcement

Family   A small stable group usually, but not always, related, and normally living together. This definition reflects the reality of family life today, and when professional workers operate according to it they are able to be less judgemental and more helpful.

Family support services (Ch. 3)   Services made available to families caring for disabled children or adults, such as child minding, day care and short-term residential care. Recognition of the need for such services reflects the awareness that families cannot and should not be expected to care for quite dependent disabled people without appropriate support services.
See also Community care

Family group home (Ch. 14)   Residential accommodation for a small group of children where helpers live in the residence and take parenting roles. The family group home model of residential care is inappropriate for adults because it subjects them to infantilising experiences, abnormal relationships and prevents age-appropriate behaviour.
See also Group residence, Infantilising lifestyle, Parenting

Fine motor skills   *See* Motor skill

Foster care   Care of children who are unable to live with their natural parents by other adults. Foster parents are accountable to helping agencies and receive a financial allowance to cover basic costs. Today's approach to the care of disabled children favours the development of foster care for short- and medium-term placement. Where separation from natural parents is permanent, adoption is preferable.
See also Adoption

Genetic   A term describing disabling conditions that are transmitted from generation to generation, for example, cystic fibrosis.

Genetic counselling   Advising people with genetic conditions of the possibilities of their condition being passed on to their children and to subsequent generations.
See also Genetic

Goals (Ch 7)   A general statement about what a specific program seeks to achieve.
See also Objectives, Programming

Gross motor skills   *See* Motor skills

Group residence (Ch 11)   A residence where a small group of disabled adults live and are assisted by helpers who may or may not live with them.
See also Community residences, Family group home, Small community residences

Habilitation   Providing a decent and beneficial way of life for disabled people previously denied it as a result of institutional living.
See also Congregate care, Deprivation, Institution, Privation, Rehabilitation

Handicap   This term is often used as an alternative to disability. There are, however, significant differences in the meanings of the two words and they should not be confused.
A disability is a functional restriction caused by some form of impairment, whereas a handicap is the consequence to disabled people of the social, emotional and physical barriers devised to exclude them from society. Handicaps therefore reside in the attitudes of others and in the physical environment.
See also Access, Disability, Impairment

Helper   An employed or voluntary worker directly or indirectly assisting disabled people.

Helping professions   Groups of helpers directly or indirectly assisting disabled people. In its more precise meaning this term refers to specific groups of helpers who have received training in disciplines such as social work, psychology, occupational therapy, etc.

Helplessness (Ch. 16)   Being unable to assist oneself because of disability, unreasonable restrictions imposed by others, inadequate and inconsistent socialisation experiences or a self-concept which emphasises dependence upon others (Seligman 1975)
A state of helplessness:
• inhibits effort, commitment and determination
• is a barrier to learning
• produces anxiety that can affect a person's sense of well-being and emotional state.
See also Self-concept

Hemiplegia   Paralysis of one side of the body as a result of some kind of damage to the central nervous system, for example, in some forms of cerebral palsy or following a stroke.

Holistic   This concept asserts that a whole is greater than the sum of its parts. A holistic approach seeks to understand disabled people as individuals, to identify and comprehend their needs in the context of their total life situation and to offer help consistent with that understanding. This approach, which is similar to interdisciplinary orientations, differs from those where helpers comprehend and respond to disabled people only from the narrowness of their particular disciplines.
See also Teamwork

Homemaker   An employed or voluntary worker assisting a disabled person living alone, a group of disabled people living together or a family caring for a disabled person. A homemaker undertakes a range of domestic and other essential daily tasks to enable the individual, group or family to function effectively, to become more independent or to prevent breakdown.
See also Attendant care

Hostel   A term describing residential facilities assisting clients at a stage before independent living. The concept of hostel accommodation is sometimes linked to the idea of a continuum of care, that is, a range of accommodation from total care to independent living. According to this idea, as clients develop skills and greater degrees of independence they should be moved from residence to residence until they are living independently. While contemporary approaches emphasise the need to increase the independence of clients, the idea of continual movement as a way of achieving it is not desirable because independent living is a right and not something to be progressively earned.
See also Least restrictive alternative

Human services   A broad term that describes all types of services provided to people in need by helping and welfare agencies in the public, charitable or private sectors.

Hydrocephaly   A condition in which there is an accumulation of cerebro-spinal fluid in the skull.

Impairment   The characteristics of the individual that cause disability, for example spinal injury, brain damage.
   See also Disability, Handicap

Incontinence   Loss of control of bowel or bladder caused mainly by physical but also sometimes by psychological factors, or by delayed development.

Independence (Ch. 2)   Being able to do as much for oneself as one is able, and not being unnecessarily dependent upon or subject to the control of others. When used in relation to disabled people this term conveys the belief that most are capable of acting independently in many aspects of their lives and so should be free from external constraint and unnecessary forms of help. The notion of independence is not only a key concept on which contemporary approaches are based, it represents a criticism of past approaches which emphasised dependence.
   See also Independent living, Infantilising lifestyle.

Independent living   Living without unnecessary or unreasonable dependence upon others. While independent living is a desirable and attainable goal for many disabled people, it is at the same time important to acknowledge that in reality almost all members of society are dependent upon others in some way, and so independent living for disabled people should not be pursued to an unreasonable extent.
   See also Independence, Least restrictive alternative

Individualisation   Treating disabled people as individuals with quite specific needs, interests, desires and preferences, and not simply as one of a category.
   See also Category

Individual plan (Ch. 5)   A plan detailing the needs of a disabled person and the ways in which some or all of those needs can be met. Individual plans are essential for most disabled people assisted in residential contexts to ensure that needs are identified and appropriate assistance provided. Whenever possible, clients should be involved in the preparation of such plans and also, where appropriate, their close relatives.

Industrialisation   *See* Industrial revolution

Industrial revolution (Ch. 1)   This term refers to major changes in social, economic and occupational aspects of society as a result of the introduction of machinery to processes of production. Industrialisation created social conditions that resulted in the movement of large numbers of disabled people into institutions
   See also Laissez-faire, Protestant ethic

Infantilising lifestyle   Subjecting disabled adolescents or adults to a lifestyle that keeps them in a child-like and dependent state. An infantilising lifestyle involves the denial of opportunities to make decisions and to experience adult roles and relationships. Many past forms of residential care can be criticised as having imposed infantilising lifestyles on disabled people.
   See also Dignity of risk, Independence

Inmate   A person who lives in any form of custodial institution.
   See also Congregate care, Institution

Institution   In a purely descriptive sense, an institution is a large residential facility. This term is, however, more frequently used in a judgemental and condemning way to describe any type of residence that controls and contains inmates and operates with a depersonalising and dehumanising regime.
   See also Congregate care, Dehumanising, Inmate, Total Institution

Institutional neurosis   On admission to institutions inmates were expected to behave entirely according to the dictates of staff. Since this necessitated accommodation to a dehumanising pattern of life, it often produced in inmates disengagement and a range of detrimental and sometimes bizarre coping mechanisms. Barton (1976: 2–3) who developed this idea, suggests institutional neurosis to be:

> characterised by apathy, lack of initiative, loss of interest more marked in things and events not immediately personal or present, submissiveness, and sometimes no expression of feelings of resentment at harsh or unfair orders. There is also a lack of interest in the future and an apparent inability to make practical plans for it, a deterioration in personal habits, toilet and standards generally, a loss of individuality, and a resigned acceptance that things will go on as they are — unchangingly, inevitably and indefinitely.

Until this pattern of behaviour in inmates was accounted for in terms of adjustment to institutional life, it was widely believed to be a natural consequence of disability or difference.
   See also Coping mechanism, Institutionalisation

Institutionalisation   The consequences of enforced institutional living for the behaviour and self-concept of the individual. The term is often used to describe people who have been depersonalised by harsh and rigid institutional regimes which have rendered them apathetic and helpless.
   See also Helplessness, Institutional neurosis

Intake system (Ch. 4)   A formally established process for responding to requests for services and allocating vacancies. Intake systems are today considered essential in ensuring that services go to those with greatest need.
   See also Allocation team

Integration   *See* Community integration

Intellectual disability   Limitations in intellectual ability that restrict the way an individual functions within society, particularly in meeting social demands and expectations. Intellectual disability can be caused by:
- damage to the brain arising from such factors as congenital defects, birth difficulties, illness or accident
- social impairment, that is, having been subjected to social experiences that have prevented intellectual development.

Four categories of intellectual disability have traditionally been used; mild, moderate, severe and profound retardation. The usual way of assigning individuals to one of these categories was by assessing their intelligence, social skills and adaptive behaviour. These categories are now beginning to lose their popularity because they serve no useful function.
   See also Adaptive behaviour, Category, Intelligence tests, Self-fulfilling prophesy, Social skills

Intelligence tests   Tests devised by psychologists which seek to measure intelligence. Such tests are no longer used to the extent they once were and, in fact, opposition to their use has reached the point where, in some North American states, their use in relation to some social groups is illegal. Among reasons for the decline in their popularity are that:

- there is now considerable doubt about the nature of intelligence
- the scores people obtain on tests vary considerably over time and on different tests, and can be increased by coaching
- many questions in tests are a measure of abilities that are not innate but which can be learned
- there is often a cultural and class bias in tests, that is, the competencies they seek to measure are those that are relevant to middle and upper socio-economic groups
- an individual's intelligence quotient tends to be used as a basis for making many unsubstantiated generalisations and judgements about him/her.

The use of intelligence tests with disabled people is objected to not only because they have made possible the location of disabled people in rigidly conceived categories, but they also reinforce negative stereotypes.

See also Assessment, Category, Classification, Stereotype

Interaction   Communication, dealings, actions between two or more people where there is give and take and mutual or reciprocal action.

Interactive learning (Ch. 8)   Using everyday interactions to ensure that clients develop skills. As clients and helpers undertake tasks together the attention of clients is directed to what they need to learn, and activities are structured to enable learning to take place. In short, interactive learning closely resembles the normal ways in which people learn.

Interdisciplinary approach   *See* Teamwork

Intermittent reinforcement   *See* Reinforcement

Interpersonal relationships   Relationships between two or more people.

Intimacy   A term describing closeness and familiarity between people and exchange of quite personal knowledge and feelings. Close friendships and most relationships within families can be described as intimate, and intimacy is a natural and essential aspect of human experience.

Intrinsic reinforcement   *See* Reinforcement

Key worker (Chs 5 & 17)   A helper who accepts responsibility for ensuring that a client receives all forms of assistance detailed in an individual plan and who provides necessary personalised care to that client.

See also Individual plan

Labelling   A concept indicating the way in which the naming of a deviant group, such as homosexuals, spastics and alcoholics, sets in motion a process that results in individuals being evaluated in terms of a negative stereotype.

See also Category, Classification, Stereotype

Laissez-faire   A term used to describe the economic philosophy which made possible the rapid development of industrialisation in the late eighteenth and early nineteenth centuries. Laissez-faire, meaning leaving alone, or non-interference, asserts that economic, business or industrial affairs operate most effectively and to the greatest benefit of all when they are entirely free from government control.

See also Industrial revolution, Liberalism

Least restrictive alternative (Ch. 2)   A principle governing the provision of services for disabled people asserting that assistance should be made available in contexts which offer the greatest degree of personal freedom. This principle is based on the belief that clients cannot be assisted if services unnecessarily deprive them of liberty or inhibit normal development and integration. Restrictions on clients should be imposed only when it is evident that their needs cannot be met in unrestricted situations or where living in such situations results in a threat to the well-being of clients or others. This principle is applied mainly to accommodation, suggesting that, wherever possible, disabled people should live in typical domestic-type situations. It does, however, have relevance for the education, work, leisure and health needs of disabled people, suggesting that these needs also should be met wherever possible in contexts typical for society.

See also Dignity of risk, Normalisation

Liberalism (Ch. 1)   A philosophy asserting that individuals are free to behave as they wish and are not bound by responsibilities and obligations to others. This philosophy became dominant in eighteenth century western Europe and today underpins the structure of most western societies. Liberalism is seen to have contributed to the destruction of the pre-industrial social order through its rejection of community-oriented values.

See also Industrialisation, Laissez-faire

Mainstream society   This term is used in the book in two ways. First, it refers to all aspects of social life beyond the traditional closed institution. Second, it refers to shared standards, beliefs, values and patterns of life within society that are supported and practised by the majority. While this is to a certain extent the case, it is important to acknowledge that the degree of commonality is not as great as is sometimes thought. A close examination of social life reveals society to be made up not of one dominant group with a small deviant minority, but a plurality of groups from different social classes, religions, ethnic backgrounds and political persuasions. While these groups together constitute society, and for the most part co-exist harmoniously, they do, in fact, support and operate according to contrasting and often opposing belief systems. It is now accepted that a pluralistic society is to be desired, not only because it is consistent with the basic values of western society, but because of the richness its diversity brings.

From the point of view of disabled people, they become, in a pluralistic society, a legitimate rather than a deviant group.

See also Abnormal, Normalisation, Pluralism

Mainstreaming (Ch. 15)   Mainstreaming describes the contemporary approach to meeting the educational needs of certain groups of disadvantaged children, particularly those who are disabled. In the past such children were educated in specialised contexts either in special classes in normal schools or in special day or residential schools.

The basic objections to such arrangements arise from the fact that not only did they not meet the educational needs of the children concerned, but they also had the function of locating them in deviant identities and a stigmatised status.

The idea of mainstreaming asserts that, wherever possible, disadvantaged children should be educated in normal schools. While there will remain a need for specialised resources for some children, mainstreaming will lead to a substantial reduction in their number. Making mainstreaming a reality entails considerable change in certain aspects of the educational system, in the organisation of school life and in teacher attitudes.

The term mainstreaming is now beginning to be used as a general concept to assert that all services for disabled people should be integrated into social life.

See also Deviants, Integration, Normalisation, Stigma

Management styles (Ch. 18)   The patterned ways in which those in senior positions in organisations deal with workers and organisational issues. There are many ways of exploring management styles; in this book they are considered in terms of directive and participative management.

See also Directive management, Participative management

Maturity   Reaching a level of development that is equated wth adulthood. It is believed that many, if not most, disabled people can become mature if given necessary assistance to develop appropriate understandings, skills and behaviour.

See also Developmental approach

Medicalisation (Ch. 1)   Dealing with people categorised as deviant, including those with disabilities, as if they were sick and in need of treatment. Objections to medicalisation are based on the fact that most deviant people are not sick; they either behave in ways that depart from what is considered to be normal or they have some form of disability or handicap. When deviant people are viewed and treated as if they are sick, they are assumed to be incapable of being responsible for themselves and to require the kinds of help medical practitioners, nurses and hospitals provide. Medical conceptions of disabled people have not served them well and should be used only when medical needs become paramount.

See also Category, Deviants, Diagnosis, Handicap, Normality, Sick role, Therapy

Microcephaly   A condition in whch the individual has an abnormally small head and incomplete development of the brain resulting in intellectual disability.

Misfits   *See* Deviants

Modelling (Ch. 8)   A way of learning behaviour associated with a social role that involves clients observing and then imitating what they have seen.

See also Demonstration

Motivation (Ch. 7)   An incentive or drive which causes a person to act in a certain way. A person can be motivated by pleasant or unpleasant stimuli orginating within or external to the individual.

See also Reinforcement

Motor skill   A skill associated with the activity of muscles, for example:

Gross motor skills: the ability to use the larger parts of the body, such as trunk legs and arms, in such basic activities as crawling, walking and climbing.

Fine motor skills: the ability to perform skills with the hands such as grasping, twisting and turning, and use of objects such as cutlery and tools.

Many disabled people have difficulty in motor skills and require specialised help or aids.

Multidisciplinary approach   *See* Teamwork

Multiple disability   Possessing more than one type of disability, for example, intellectual physical, sensory disability.

Need (Ch. 6)   Something which is necessary to enable an individual to function satisfactorily. Need can be determined by both subjective and objective criteria.

Negotiation (Ch. 10)   The process that enables individuals and groups to discuss and resolve their differences. When applied to residential life, the concept of negotiation serves to indicate that since clients and helpers often desire different ends, they need to discuss and negotiate to agree on mutually acceptable courses of action. The method by which differences were resolved in the past, by managers imposing their decisions on direct care workers and by those workers imposing them on clients, is inconsistent with contemporary approaches to disabled people and the management of helping organisations.

See also Consensus decision making, Non-authoritarian, Participative management

Non-authoritarian   This term is used to describe individuals who relate to and deal with others, not from an unquestioned assumption about the correctness of their own beliefs and actions, but from an awareness that people see issues differently and seek different ends. The non-authoritarian individual respects others in terms of their differences in beliefs and values and is willing and able to enter into processes of negotiation to resolve contentious issues. While this term, like its opposite, authoritarian, is highly problematic, it nevertheless has value in explaining the behaviour of individuals, particularly those in positions of responsibility in organisations.

See also Authoritarian, Directive management, Negotiation, Participative management

Normalisation (Ch. 2)   The concept of normalisation asserts that disabled people are, as members of society, no different from others and so should have access to the opportunities and patterns of life typical for a society, together with accompanying rights and freedoms.

See also Abnormal, Normalised environment, Normality

Normalised environment   Ensuring that the living environment for disabled people is as normal as possible, that is, having taken into account any specialised needs arising from disability and having met them, providing a context for daily life that is not basically different from that of other members of society.

See also Dignity of risk, Least restrictive alternative, Normalisation, Normality

Normality   Despite the variety of ways in which the helping professions use this term, when it is applied to individuals it involves judgements of them according to specific and often idealised beliefs about wholeness and acceptability. Notions of normality vary considerably from society to society, within a society and often from one generation to another.

See also Abnormal, Mainstream society, Normalisation

Nuclear family　The small family unit comprising a parent or parents and children living in a single residence. The wider family, which includes other close relatives, is known as the extended family.

See also Family

Nurturing　Bringing up and caring for children in an attentive and concerned way so that their basic needs are met.

Objectives (Ch. 7)　When used in the context of programming, objectives are precise, action-based statements as to what a program sets out to achieve.

See also Goals, Programming

Observation　Watching how a client copes with the everyday aspects of life, or when attempting to perform a specific task, in order to gain an understanding that can serve as a basis for the provision of assistance.

See also Assessment

Occupational therapist　A trained helper who provides specialised assistance to develop or maintain the typical activities of daily life.

Organisation-centred approach　The way in which the dominant patterns and traditions of an organisation or residence serve no purpose other than maintaining the day-to-day operation of that organisation or residence. Where this occurs in residential settings the needs of client are seldom taken into account and rarely met.

See also Client-centred approach, Staff-centred approach, Tradition-centred approach

Paraplegia　Paralysis of the lower part of the body, often caused by injury to the spinal cord in the region of the central or lower back.

Parenting (Ch. 14)　A term describing the functions and responsibilities of natural parents which should be assumed by direct care workers when assisting children in residential contexts.

Parkinson's disease　A condition associated with disease or damage to a specific part of the brain. It may cause the person affected to develop rigidity in body, a stooping posture, a shuffling walk, to lose control of facial expression and head movement and experience difficulty in speech.

Participative management (Ch. 18)　A way of managing workers based on the belief that their involvement in decision-making, particularly decisions likely to affect them in any way, is essential. Once workers do become involved in decision-making an entirely new pattern of worker–management relationships develops. Research suggests participative management to be highly successful in organisations where conditions are continually changing, where the means of achieving the organisation's goals are integral to ends sought and where workers expect to obtain considerable job satisfaction. Participative management is considered to be the only way organisations providing assistance to disabled people can be successfully managed.

See also Directive management

Peonage (Ch. 15)　Originally this term referred to the practice of keeping debtors or convicts in a subservient state to work off debts or make amends for their crimes. It aptly describes the situation of many disabled people in residential accommodation and day centres today because they continue to be compelled to work and without income. To use them as a form of cheap labour to maintain a residence or output is now seen as abusive. Disabled people, like others, should be able to choose whether they work, and when they do, to receive adequate reward.

Perceptions　The process by which individuals become aware of something in their environment as a result of stimulation of the senses.

This term is often coupled with the word selective to indicate that individuals develop set ways of perceiving the world around them as a result of personal life experiences, interests and beliefs.

When the concept of selective perception is applied to disabled people it reveals the processes operating within society by which they have come to be understood as inadequate and abnormal. In brief, most non-disabled people have grown up within a society that holds quite specific and negative views of disabled people and, without realising it, have automatically taken on those views as their own. One of the tasks of people assisting disabled members of society is to work to change those perceptions.

See also Deviants, Self-fulfilling prophesy

Personal dignity　An individual's sense of worth, value, humanness and uniqueness that develops and is maintained mainly as a result of the way others communicate appropriate regard, respect and concern.

See also Self-concept

Personal social service organisations　Organisations providing services directly to people in need. Personal social service organisations incude those assisting children and families, young offenders, aged and disabled people, and are usually staffed by social and welfare workers.

Phenylketonuria (PKU)　An hereditary disorder which affects the nervous system as a result of the failure of the body to produce an enzyme to deal with the amino-acid phenylalanine. The condition can be detected following birth and brain damage prevented by a low phenylalanine diet.

Physiotherapist　A trained helper who specialises in treating clients with illnesses and conditions, especially those where motor functioning has been impaired, by means of heat, massage and exercise.

Plan co-ordinators　*See* Case manager

Pluralism　An analysis of society which suggests it to comprise, not one major group with common beliefs, values and patterns of behaviour, but many social groupings with different and often competing beliefs, values and behaviour. Most western societies are said to be pluralistic, and pluralism is now seen to be desirable because of the richness and variety it brings to social life. Pluralism implies toleration of individual difference, and, for disabled people, full membership of society and integration into social life.

See also Abnormal, Mainstream society, Normality

Poor laws (Ch. 1)   Laws relating to the control of and assistance to all classes of poor, including orphaned children, destitute families, unemployed, sick and disabled people. The most famous, or perhaps infamous, poor laws were introduced in Britain in the early part of the nineteenth century and led to the development of a vast system of institutions known as workhouses. Under these laws, admission to a workhouse was the only way an individual or family could obtain assistance from the state. To prevent people from remaining in the workhouse, everything about its pattern of life was made deliberately harsh and unpleasant.
See also Workhouse

Positive discrimination   Taking action to ensure that disabled people are favoured in preference to others when allocating funds, establishing programs or making decisions about their education, work and leisure needs. It is argued that it is only by discriminating positively in their favour that the neglect and ill-treatment of the past can be corrected, and disabled people become fully integrated and participating members of society.
See also Discrimination

Presenting needs   When an individual, group or family seeks help, certain needs are immediately apparent. Often, however, some of these presenting needs, while being real, are less important than others still to be identified. It is thus necessary for helpers to ensure that they have an adequate understanding of client need before taking action, and that they are not just responding to presenting needs.
See also Need

Pre-placement program (Ch. 4)   A program detailing the ways in which particular clients and those close to them should be prepared for residential placement.
See also Programming

Pressure group   An organised group of people who act on their own behalf or on behalf of others to obtain greater recognition or increased services. Pressure groups typically produce information, lobby politicians and governments and use the media to promote their cause. Because of the nature of the political systems in western societies, there is often a close relationship between the effectiveness of pressure groups and services provided to the people on whose behalf they act. Many voluntary bodies assisting disabled people operate as pressure groups.
See also Advocacy

Priority systems (Ch. 4)   Where services for disabled people are insufficient, it is necessary to establish priority systems to ensure that services go to those with greatest need.

Privacy (Ch. 10)   Being able to get away from others and be alone in both a physical and psychological sense. Life in many residential settings renders privacy impossible because of the congregate nature of care. It is now argued that since privacy is so important to the personal dignity and self-identity of the individual, the operation of residential facilities should be modified in whatever ways are necessary to enable clients to experience and enjoy the degree of privacy other members of society enjoy.

Privation   Denial of the usual comforts of life considered essential for normal emotional growth and social functioning.
See also Congregate care, Dehumanising, Depersonalising lifestyle, Deprivation, Total institution

Problem people   *See* Deviants

Program evaluation (Ch. 7)   Systematic examination of a program to determine the extent to which its goals and objectives have been achieved.
See also Goals, Objectives, Programming

Program objectives   *See also* Objectives

Programming (Ch. 7)   Any systematically organised, implemented and evaluated process oriented to some form of help. In this book this term is mostly used in a somewhat narrower way to refer to forms of help for developing specific client skills. Essentially, this kind of behavioural programming involves close analysis of behaviour or skills clients are to learn, assessing their ability to perform that behaviour or skill and presenting to them, in a planned sequence, the various aspects of what they need to learn.

Progressive   A term used to describe certain disabilities to indicate that they are increasing in severity, bringing about greater disability, and probably, directly or indirectly, resulting in earlier death.
See also Degenerative

Prompting (Ch. 7)   Prompting refers to the way in which cues are given to clients to enable them to become aware of the next action they have to perform in learning a specific behaviour.

Protestant ethic (Ch. 1)   A set of beliefs, considered to have resulted from Protestant interpretations of Biblical ideas, asserting that work is divinely ordained, a natural and necessary activity and an end in itself rather than simply a means to an end. It is argued that the Protestant ethic legitimised the economic system that made possible large scale nineteenth century industrialisation by creating a belief that the individual had a duty to work. The dominance of the Protestant ethic in industrialised societies has meant that those who would not or could not work, including disabled people, were negatively regarded.
See also Industrial revolution, Liberalism.

Psychiatrist   A medically trained worker who specialises in the study and treatment of mental and emotional disorders.

Psychologist   A trained worker who attempts to understand the cognitive, affective, behavioural and social functioning of people in order to assess needs and develop helping approaches.

Punishment (Ch. 16)   Imposing some form of penalty on an individual because his/her behaviour has been judged to be unacceptable.

Quadraplegia   Paralysis of lower parts of the body involving the trunk and parts of both arms. Quadraplegia is often caused by injury to the spinal cord in the region of the neck.

Reciprocity   Give and take between people where there is mutual benefit.

Records (Ch. 9)   Helping disabled people in residential settings, however normalised those settings, is a relatively formal process undertaken by organisations. Helpers involved are required to maintain a range of records relating to the assistance they provide and the general operation of residences. Records are important for purposes of accountability.

See also Accountability, Client records

Reference group   Groups that individuals identify with, and whose standards and behaviour they use as a basis for evaluating and establishing their own values, beliefs and behaviour. Individuals often have different reference groups for different dimensions of their lives.

Regionally-based services (Ch. 3)   The planning and provision of services on a regional, district or area basis and in a decentralised way.

See also Centrally-based services

Rehabilitation   Provision of help to individuals who have become disabled to enable them to recover, to the maximum extent possible, their original skills. This term is often used to suggest the provision of services to compensate for deprivations experienced by people who have spent the whole of their lives in institutions. The appropriate term for this process is habilitation.

See also Habilitation

Reinforcement (Ch. 8)   An event or object that increases, maintains or reduces certain behaviour. Reinforcement can be:

- positive, designed to encourage behaviour
- negative, designed to discourage behaviour
- intrinsic, providing satisfaction as a result of behaving in the desired way
- extrinsic, providing satisfaction as a result of some kind of reward.

Residual welfare function   Provision of help by the state to people in need only when they can demonstrate that they are unable to help themselves and cannot obtain help from voluntary and charitable agencies. It is argued today that many groups of disadvantaged people, particularly disabled, have a right to adequate assistance whenever they are in need and not when all else fails.

See also Blaming the victim

Respite care   Providing temporary relief for those who care full-time at home for a disabled child or adult by means of residential accommodation. Used well, respite care can also benefit clients by providing them with a break from their usual pattern of life, opportunities to meet new people and to learn new skills. While this form of care is necessary, the choice of the term respite has somewhat unfortunate connotations for disabled people in that it implies temporary relief of suffering, thereby suggesting that disabled people are the cause of the suffering experienced by their carers. For this reason a more appropriate term is short-term care.

See also Short-term care

Rights (Ch. 2)   The basic standards to which an individual is entitled and which are recognised and protected under law.

Ritual   Doing something in a set and unalterable way. When a task becomes ritualised it tends to be carried out in the set way not because of what is achieves but for its own sake. Often rituals are so central to the life of a group of people or an organisation that it is considered unthinkable to question them. Rituals play a significant part in the daily life of many residential facilities and they bind both clients and direct care workers to certain courses of behaviour. Almost any dimension of everyday life can become ritualised, for example, the way beds are made, the time of bed making, placement of clothes in a cupboard, the way washing up is done, teeth cleaning. Not only do such rituals make no real sense, they tend to depersonalise by subjecting clients to identical and meaningless experiences regardless of individual preference or need.

Role (Ch. 8)   Rights, expectations and duties that accompany positions people occupy in society. One person in the course of the day becomes involved in many roles and he/she is expected to behave appropriately in each. A male adult may, for example, be involved in the roles of father, husband, driver, colleague, committee member. It is clear that functioning effectively in society involves a relatively accurate awareness of the behaviour accompanying roles and being able to perform that behaviour appropriately. It is argued that unless disabled people are encouraged to perform different roles and are able to function in them with some degree of success, they will never achieve the desired degree of integration.

See also Role play, Role reversal, Sick role

Role play (Ch. 8)   A way of enabling an individual to learn behaviour associated with a particular role by acting that role in a specially structured learning situation.

See also Role, Role reversal

Role reversal (Ch. 8)   Acting the role of another person in order to learn and better appreciate what that role entails both for the individual in the role and those interacting with him/her.

See also Role, Role play

Routine (Ch. 10)   The patterned way in which something is undertaken and accomplished. The most obvious routine is the daily routine which, for disabled people living in residential accommodation, is often rigidly structured to meet staff convenience, achieved by controlling every aspect of the client's day and imposed on clients irrespective of their needs or wishes. Contemporary approaches emphasise flexible client-centred and client-determined routines

See also Client-centred approach, Ritual

Segregation   Keeping disabled people unnecessarily physically, socially and emotionally isolated from society by using special residential, educational, work, leisure and health facilities.

See also Mainstreaming

Self-concept   The individual's perception of himself/herself. Self-concept is significantly shaped and influenced as a result of the way others value and treat the individual. It is argued that many disabled people have low self-concepts because of their lack of value in the eyes of others. Their self-concept can be enhanced by ensuring that they have the means to function as normal members of society and to influence the world around them to their own advantage.

Self-fulfilling prophesy   Where an individual, group or society believes something to be true, they tend to organise their perceptions in a way that confirms those beliefs. Where, for example, workers in a residential setting believe adult disabled people to be little different from children, they interpret their behaviour according to that belief. This often causes clients to behave in inappropriate ways, so confirming and reinforcing beliefs of helpers.

This concept has considerable significance in explaining how disabled people have come to be trapped by quite false definitions of their capabilities and their place in society.

See also Perceptions

Self-help group A group of people with similar concerns, problems and difficulties who assist one another. Self-help groups may include groups of disabled people or groups of parents, relatives and friends. Sometimes helpers assist self-help groups but only to the extent that they wish to be assisted. Self-help groups also act as pressure groups.

See also Advocacy, Pressure group

Service delivery (Ch. 3) Arrangements by which organisations providing services make them available to clients.

Shaping (Ch. 7) A technique used in structured programming, particularly behaviour modification programs, which involves reinforcing approximations of a desired behaviour in a way that, over a period of time, leads to precise performance of that behaviour.

See also Programming

Shared living *See* Democratic living

Sheltered workshop A day centre where disabled people are trained for work in open employment or where they remain working in a protected environment. Sheltered workshops usually undertake contract work involving light assembly and packing.

See also Adult training centre, Day care services

Short-term care Residential accommodation provided on a limited basis, not exceeding six weeks. Usually short-term care is planned in order to meet the particular needs of a client or those with whom he/she lives.

See also Emergency care, Respite care

Sick role When individuals become sick they are treated in a new and quite different way, that is, they are expected to set aside their present roles and responsibilities and take on the role of sick person. There are clear expectations associated with the sick role, (Parsons, 1951) including:

- accepting that you are sick and wanting to get better
- recognising your need for treatment
- complying with instructions given by those responsible for your treatment.

As a result of the use of medical approaches, disabled people have been treated as if they were sick. This has meant that they have become, because of the permanency of most disabling conditions, located for life in sick roles and as sick people. It is today asserted that, disability is not a sickness and so disabled people should not be dealt with as if they were sick.

See also Diagnosis, Medicalisation, Role, Therapy

Small community residences (Ch. 11) A house or flat in the community in which a group of not more than six disabled people live. Such residences are usually purchased or rented by helping organisations for this purpose, or rented by groups of clients themselves. The development of small community residences is advocated because such residences are seen to afford the greatest possibilities for a normal life.

Social role *See* Role

Social skills Skills necessary for interacting with others and functioning in society.

Social worker A trained worker who seeks to assist clients on a personal, interpersonal or social level.

Socialisation The process by which an individual acquires the perceptions, beliefs, and patterns of behaviour shared by a group or a society. Traditionally, two forms of socialisation have been recognised: primary socialisation, which is achieved as a result of a child's interactions within the family in the early years, and secondary socialisation which occurs in such contexts as school, work and other social groupings.

See also Perceptions, Role

Social philosophy Beliefs about the ways in which social life should be ordered and individual relationships structured. It would seem evident that conceptions and treatment of disabled people are closely related to the dominant social philosophy of a society.

Spastic Spasticity refers to the tightening of muscles so that movement is inhibited. The term spastic relates to one particular form of cerebral palsy but tends to be used as a label for all cerebral palsied people.

See also Cerebral palsy, Labelling

Speech pathologist A trained worker who assists clients in language development or who helps those whose communication has been impaired by injury or disease.

Spina bifida A congenital condition involving malformation of the backbone. This results in inadequate protection for the spinal cord which protrudes and often leads to paralysis.

Staff-centred approach The way in which the dominant patterns and traditions within an organisation or residence are structured to meet the needs of staff. In such contexts the needs of clients are rarely met.

See also Client-centred approach, Organisation-centred approach, Tradition-centred approach

State as parent The belief, enacted in law, that the state should assume responsibility for people deemed incapable of providing for or protecting themselves. This notion has been applied extensively to disabled adults, and while having certain beneficial consequences, has also operated contrary to their interests in that it has reinforced the view that they were like children and therefore in need of protection.

See also Infantilising lifestyle

Stereotype A set of preconceived, over-simplified and often erroneous beliefs about individuals or groups. Stereotypes are usually maintained despite evidence to the contrary and feature significantly in reinforcing deviant conceptions of disabled people.

See also Category, Classification, Labelling, Self-fulfilling prophesy

Stigma   Originally this term described a mark placed on an individual's body to denote outcast or slave. More recently it has been used about anything visible that can be identified with deviance. Often efforts to help disabled people through the provision of special resources, facilities and equipment have served to stigmatise, and even residential accommodation is felt to be stigmatising.

Stress (Ch. 19)   The effects of demands on an individual's sense of well-being, physiological state and relationships with which he/she cannot cope.

Support services   Services to enable clients and those assisting them to achieve adequate care, a reasonable standard of life or greater independence. Support services are either taken to clients and their families at home or made available in the community.

Task analysis (Ch. 7)   Breaking down a task or skill into its many skill components. Task analysis can provide an assessment of an individual's present performance and highlight where the person is having difficulty in learning.

Teaching approaches (Ch. 8)   Ways in which a disabled person can be assisted to acquire skills.

Teamwork (Ch. 19)   Teamwork is achieved when a group of workers collaborate to achieve goals that individuals cannot achieve when acting alone. Teamwork is essential in residential contexts where groups of helpers are providing assistance to groups of clients.

When workers from differing helping professions are involved in assisting specific clients, the traditional approach has been a *multi-disciplinary* one. Such an approach involves workers assisting clients according to the beliefs and practices of their individual professions. While workers are aware that other professionals have a contribution to make, they do not identify a need for close collaboration.

Contemporary approaches see a need for interdisciplinary and transdisciplinary orientations. An *interdisciplinary approach* involves considerable collaboration among differing professionals in pursuit of uniformity and consistency. *Transdisciplinary* approaches, on the other hand, are based upon the need for those workers assisting a client to arrive at a common understanding of the ways in which he/she should be assisted. There is considerable sharing of roles and functions, and often a key worker acts on behalf of others in providing assistance to the client.

See also Key worker

Therapeutic community   A residential environment, orginally developed in the context of the psychiatric hospital, where the daily life of the community and the interactions of members, including staff, are a major dimension of treatment. The pattern of life in a therapeutic community includes democracy in decision-making and the absence of rigid distinctions between clients and helpers.

Therapy   The process used to treat a medical condition. When used in work with disabled people, therapy refers to assistance provided by those with medical or clinical training. Since therapy is oriented to the cure of disease, it is perhaps an inappropriate term to use when assisting disabled people because most do not have diseases that can be cured. Furthermore, the term therapy is often

attached to quite meaningless activities in order to render them plausible. The term is probably best avoided unless it refers to a process that focuses on treatment of a condition which can be classified as an illness or disease. After all, the daily activities of non-disabled people are not called therapy. Whenever the term is used unnecessarily it serves to reinforce the belief that disabled people are sick.

See also Diagnosis, Medicalisation, Sick role, Treatment.

Time out   A technique used in behaviour modification programs which involves removing the person from situations which are reinforcing undesirable behaviour. The person is placed in a context that offers nothing that interests or stimulates him/her and is not dealt with in a way that might reinforce his/er undesirable behaviour.

See also Behaviour modification

Total institution   A form of congregate care where inmates are cut off from the wider society, where all activities and aspects of the day are carried out within one setting and where every facet of the lives of inmates is subject to the control of people with authority over them. Most forms of congregate care were, in the past, total institutions (Goffman, 1961).

See also Congregate care, Depersonalising lifestyle, Institution, Institutional neurosis, Institutionalisation

Tradition-centred approach   The way in which the significant aspects of the operation of a residence become structured by tradition. Daily life in such a context makes little sense when explored in terms of staff or client need; it simply operates in a ritualised way because that is the way it has always operated.

See also Client-centred approach, Organisation-centred approach, Ritual, Tradition-centred approach

Transdisciplinary approach   *See* Teamwork

Treatment   A term similar in meaning to therapy when used about processes designed to cure or assist someone who is sick. The term, however, tends to be used in a much more generalised way to describe any form of help given to disabled people.

See also Medicalisation, Sick role, Therapy

Urbanisation   Growth in towns and an urban way of life as a result of large scale factory production.

See also Industrial revolution

Utilitarianism   A social philosophy, popular in the nineteenth century, asserting that the goal of a society should be the greatest happiness of the greatest number. Where such a philosophy serves as the basis for legislation, it follows that there is likely to be a disadvantaged minority. This philosophy significantly influenced much nineteenth century legislation and served to justify the identification of deviant groups and negative treatment of them.

Value system   Sets of beliefs shared by individuals and groups concerning aspects of social life and the way people should behave.

Voluntary agencies   Organisations providing assistance to people in need that obtain all or a significant part of their revenue from non-government sources.

See also Charities

Volunteer (Ch. 13)   An individual who offers his/her time and skills to provide assistance that will, directly or indirectly, benefit clients. No payment is made to a volunteer apart from reimbursement of minor expenses.

Waiting list (Ch. 4) Where there is an insufficiency in a service for all needing it, an effectively controlled waiting list ensures that vacancies go to those clients with greatest need.

See also Priorities

Warehousing A term used to describe the way in which large groups of deviant people, including disabled people, have been contained in institutions without any purpose or meaning beyond containment. Institutions of this kind have been likened to warehouses whose sole function is to contain objects (Miller and Gwynne, 1972).

See also Total institution, Institution, Congregate care

Welfare state A broad term describing the way in which a society, through its governments, accepts respon-

sibility for assisting people in need. Where a country has no welfare system, individuals have to fend for themselves as best they can or rely on charity. The idea of a welfare state reflects the belief that individual misfortune is the responsibility not only of the individual concerned but also of society, and so the individual has a basic entitlement to have at least his/her more important needs met by society.

See also Residual welfare function

Work ethic   *See* Protestant ethic

Workhouse (Ch. 1)   A public institution provided for the maintenance of paupers. Workhouses have existed for hundreds of years and were finally phased out earlier this century.

See also Poor law, Stigma

Questions for helpers

This section contains sets of questions which helpers and clients can use to explore the quality of residential services and the pattern of life in a particular residence. Each question has been worded to suggest an affirmative answer to be the one that is most consistent with contemporary approaches to disabled people. Where a question is answered negatively, before concluding something to be wrong, it is essential to consider the assumptions implied by the question. It may be that the helpers and clients involved do not support those assumptions and so the question will not be valid. Where, on the other hand, an answer is in the negative and the assumptions are supported, those involved may find it helpful to consider what changes or additional resources are necessary to achieve the practice in question.

BASIC PHILOSOPHY AND APPROACH

1. Do clients have the same basic rights and freedoms as other members of society?
2. Are clients viewed as being capable of growth and development?
3. Is the residence free from practices that impose infantilising lifestyles on adult clients?
4. Are clients treated as people rather than as patients?
5. Are clients encouraged to control their lives and make choices?
6. Are clients free to come and go as they wish?
7. Are client lifestyles and the pattern of life in the residence consistent with the principle of normalisation?
8. Is the residence integrated into the community?
9. Are all clients living in contexts that are the least restrictive?
10. Is the residence free from derogatory labels and demeaning names for clients?
11. Do helpers work to change negative social attitudes towards disabled people?
12. Do helpers work to ensure that the pattern of life in the residence is client centred?

PLANNING SERVICES

1. Is the assistance offered by the residence part of an overall and coherent plan of services?
2. Are services available to people in their own localities?
3. Are a number of approaches used when identifying the needs of clients?

4. Have the needs of clients in a particular locality been surveyed?
5. Are comprehensive services available to clients and their families, and not just residential care?
6. Does the residence have a clear understanding of the specific forms of assistance it should be providing to clients?
7. Is the period of time a client lives in the residence related to his/her needs?
8. Does the residence have all necessary resources, such as staff and equipment, to meet the needs of clients?
9. Does the residence provide clients and their close relatives with a clear statement of services offered?
10. Have the helpers in the residence documented what they define as good practice?

INTAKE

1. Does the residence operate with a formally documented intake process?
2. Is that process followed when the residence is requested to admit a client?
3. Does the residence admit only clients whose needs have been acknowledged by an intake meeting?
4. Are direct care workers and clients involved in intake meetings?
5. Where a waiting list exists for the residence, is it managed effectively?
6. Are the needs of those on a waiting list for residential services prioritised?
7. Is there a rational and effective way of dealing with emergency requests for admission?
8. Does the residence prepare preplacement programs for clients?
9. Is the reception of a client on the day of admission appropriately planned and undertaken?
10. Is special attention paid to clients in their first few weeks' stay in the residence?

INDIVIDUAL PLANNING

1. Do all helpers understand what is meant by individual planning?
2. Are attempts being made to introduce individual planning to the residence?
3. Is a teamwork and interdisciplinary approach taken to individual planning?
4. Is a holistic approach taken to client planning?
5. Are clients, appropriate relatives and direct care helpers involved in individual planning?
6. Are helpers developing the necessary skills to implement the recommendations of planning meetings?
7. Does the residence have designated helpers responsible for plans such as plan co-ordinators and key workers?
8. Do plans reflect all the needs of clients?
9. Are plans reviewed at regular intervals?
10. Is individual planning phased out when it is no longer necessary for particular clients?
11. Are client plans adequately documented?
12. Is a rational process used for making decisions about concluding residential placement?
13. Are programs developed to ensure that when clients leave a residence all appropriate help is provided?

IDENTIFYING AND ASSESSING NEED

1. Is assessment individualised?
2. Do the methods of assessment used in the residence identify needs that can and should be met?
3. Are clients involved in their assessment?
4. Are direct care workers involved in assessment?
5. Is use made of existing information when assessing client need?
6. Where relevant, does assessment for clients examine their needs and skills in relation to:
   • health

- family situation
- mobility and transport
- personal development and self-identity
- education
- community integration
- self-help
- communication
- vocation and work
- leisure
- daily living?

7. Do clients see and have explained the results of assessment?
8. Are the results of particular forms of assessment used in ways that are of benefit to clients?

PROGRAMMING

1. Do all helpers understand what is meant by programming?
2. Are programs consistent with client need?
3. Where relevant, are attempts being made to introduce programming?
4. Where relevant, are programs in the following areas being considered:
   - personal care
   - mobility
   - self-awareness and self-concept
   - group living
   - functioning in mainstream society
   - leisure, recreation and creativity?
5. Do clients make decisions about the programs in which they will become involved?
6. Is all necessary help given to helpers who are responsible for programs?

CLIENT RECORDS

1. Are client records kept?
2. Are records available to all who have a need to see them, including clients and their close relatives?
3. Are records relevant to a client's situation?
4. Do records contain only information that presents a balanced picture of clients?
5. Are records kept up to date?

THE RESIDENCE AS HOME

1. Are attempts made to ensure that the residential environment is as home-like as possible?
2. Do clients consider the living environment to be like home?
3. In being home-like, is the pattern of life similar to that enjoyed by other members of society?
4. Is a family model of home, with direct care workers in controlling positions, seen as inappropriate for adult disabled people?
5. Is the residence free from signs or plaques or any other features that render it abnormal?

PRIVACY

1. Are helpers aware of the importance of privacy in the lives of clients?
2. Are helpers aware of the negative consequences to clients when there are insufficient opportunities for privacy?
3. Do helpers appreciate differences in the extent to which individual clients desire privacy?
4. If there are insufficient opportunities for privacy, are steps being taken to increase them?
5. Are there places in a residence or times of the day for clients to enjoy privacy?
6. Where bedrooms are shared, is there sufficient bedspace to enable clients to enjoy appropriate levels of privacy?
7. Do clients enjoy the maximum degree of privacy when showering, bathing, dressing and using the toilet?
8. Do all members of staff and other clients knock and wait for the appropriate response before entering a client's room?
9. Are clients consulted and is their approval sought before visits by outsiders take place?
10. Are clients encouraged to respect each others' privacy?
11. Do helpers, both personally and on a

group level, keep confidences about clients?

12. Are clients able to meet with relatives and friends without the presence or uninvited intrusion of helpers?
13. Can clients have privacy in personal relationships with their own or the opposite sex?
14. Do clients have privacy when they use the telephone?
15. Is clients' mail, both inward and outward, free from staff prying and censorship?

PHYSICAL ENVIRONMENT

1. Are clients and direct care workers involved in the selection of furnishings?
2. Are furnishings home-like?
3. Is there appropriate variation in decor, e.g. walls, curtains, bed covers, lighting?
4. Does each client have a place to keep his/her belongings?
5. Is the residence kept in a good state of repair?
6. Can clients personalise their own rooms?
7. Are there appropriate dining, bathing and toileting facilities?
8. Is the facility close enough to necessary community services, for example, shops, libraries, post offices, banks, churches, sport and other recreational facilities?
9. Is the residence equipped with appropriate labour-saving devices?
10. Are all necessary aids available to clients and staff?

DIGNITY OF RISK

1. Do helpers understand the idea of dignity of risk?
2. Do helpers operate in ways that permit clients to face appropriate risk situations?
3. Do helpers assist clients in developing skills so that they can encounter and cope with risk situations?

4. Is dignity of risk applied to relationships?
5. Are all necessary attempts made to ensure that the living environment is not abnormally or unnecessarily protective?
6. For those clients for whom it is necessary, is dignity of risk developed in a gradual way?
7. Do helpers operate to prevent clients being in risk situations with which they cannot cope and which are likely to be a substantial danger to them?

SHARED LIVING

1. Do staff make every effort to consult with clients and involved them in decision-making within the residence?
2. Are clients involved in decision-making processes by means of participation in:
   - discussion groups
   - client meetings
   - client–staff meetings
   - program planning meetings
   - case conferences?
3. Are clients informed about decisions which affect them but in which they have had no involvement?
4. Are clients and helpers encouraged to get together to resolve problems as they occur?
5. Are representative client groups recognised for formal negotiations?
6. Are clients involved in making decisions about:
   - their clothing
   - menu planning
   - smoking and alcohol
   - spending their money
   - their choice of friends
   - hobbies and recreation
   - hairstyles
   - trips and holidays
   - chores
   - religious observance?
7. Are clients involved in decisions about new clients and staff?

HEALTH

1. Where clients wish to, are they free to choose their own general practitioner and dentist?
2. Do clients have access to general practitioners or dentists whenever they want?
3. Do clients know how to obtain medical advice and help?
4. Are visits to general practitioners and dentists arranged individually?
5. Are obvious health problems receiving all necessary attention?
6. Is the residence free from standards and practices which might be a threat to the health of clients?
7. Are helpers familiar with the medical needs of clients?
8. Are drugs used only as prescribed?
9. Do clients understand why they are prescribed drugs and are they aware of any side-effects?
10. Are those clients with sufficient ability to do so able to look after and administer their own medication?
11. Does a residence, or the units within a residence, have a well-maintained first aid box?
12. Do helpers know what to do in the usual kinds of domestic emergencies?
13. Are helpers able to recognise seizures and deal with them?
14. Do clients receive necessary professional assistance, for example:
    - physiotherapy
    - occupational therapy
    - audiological services?
15. Are clients familiar with the range of physical aids and equipment that may improve their mobility and lifestyle?
16. Are clients and helpers effectively assisted in the use of aids?
17. Are clients helped to reduce avoidable incontinence?
18. Are the methods used to assist incontinent clients both decent and appropriate?

RELIGIOUS AND SPIRITUAL NEEDS

1. Is there adequate recognition of the spiritual needs of clients?
2. Are staff aware of their own belief systems, and have they thought through the extent to which they have relevance for clients?
3. Are helpers free from unreasonable bias in relation to religious beliefs?
4. Are clients free to follow and practise their own faith?
5. Are all necessary supports provided within the residence and beyond it to enable clients to follow their faith?
6. Are clients who are not religious free from any impositions in relation to religious observance?
7. Is consideration and respect shown towards spiritual values so as to generate open attitudes towards religion?
8. Are ministers of religion encouraged to visit the residence and see individual clients if the clients so wish?

SAFETY

1. Do clients know what to do in the event of a fire?
2. Where appropriate, are fire drills held regularly?
3. Can clients deal with small outbreaks of fire?
4. Do clients know how to use electrical appliances such as hot plates, oven, iron, washing machine?
5. Are poisonous objects and liquids kept in appropriate containers, correctly labelled and safely stored?
6. Are clients taught to recognise dangerous or hazardous objects in the residence?
7. Are clients taught to use hazardous objects such as sharp knives and scissors?
8. Are clients able to dispose of hazardous objects such as broken glass?
9. Can clients use the phone for assistance in emergencies?

10. Do clients have the necessary skills to ensure their safety when functioning outside the residence?
11. Do clients know whom to contact and how, when an emergency occurs away from the residence?

CLIENTS' CLOTHING

1. Are clients able to possess and wear their own clothing?
2. Are clients able to wear what they like?
3. Do clients have sufficient clothes for different occasions and seasonal changes?
4. Are clients taught and encouraged to select their own clothing?
5. Do clients know their own sizes?
6. Are clients given appropriate assistance, when required, in relation to styles, fashion and colours that suit them?
7. Are clients able, with appropriate assistance, to purchase their own clothes from shops in the community?
8. Are clients assisted to acquire the necessary skills to care for their own clothes?
9. Are the necessary facilities available for clients to care for their clothes, for example, washing machine, dryer, iron?
10. If clients are unable to care for their clothes, are they kept in good condition by helpers?
11. For the client needing it, is there a member of staff who takes a personal interest in his/her clothes?
12. Do clothes worn by clients enhance their appearance?
13. Is there sufficient space for clients to store their clohtes?
14. Do clients have unrestricted access to their clothes?
15. If labelling of clothes is necessary, is the label both attractive and inconspicuous?

PERSONAL HYGIENE, GROOMING AND APPEARANCE

1. Are there on-going opportunities for clients to learn to care for themselves, for example:
   - toileting
   - washing and bathing
   - hygiene
   - hair care
   - menstrual hygiene
   - shaving?
2. Do clients have their own towels and soap?
3. Do clients have their own toothbrushes and toothpaste?
4. Do clients have their own toiletries, shampoo and other hair care equipment?
5. Is a client able to decide the regularity of bathing and showering?
6. Where helpers assist clients with hygiene, grooming or appearance, do they show respect and consideration?
7. Is the client taught how to maximise his/her personal appearance?
8. Is the client encouraged to choose a hair-style that:
   - is of his/her own liking
   - suits his/her general appearance
   - is fashionable?
9. Are clients able to attend hairdressers in the community?
10. Are female clients taught to wear consmetics and jewellery and are they able to do so?

PERSONAL POSSESSIONS

1. Do clients have a secure place to keep their personal possessions and to which they alone have access?
2. Are clients, within reason, free to have whatever possessions they desire?
3. Do clients have unrestricted access to the place where they keep their possessions?

4. Are clients free to arrange and display their possessions in whatever way they wish in their rooms or personal bedspace?
5. Are all gifts to clients treated as their personal possessions?
6. Do clients know appropriate ways of sharing, lending and borrowing?
7. Do clients have age-appropriate possessions such as:
   - money
   - toys and games
   - books, magazines and comics
   - toiletries and cosmetics
   - jewellery
   - hobby materials
   - radios and other electrical equipment
   - photographs of personal significance
   - sports equipment
   - necessary means of transport, e.g. own wheelchair?
8. Have all reasonable steps been take to prevent theft?
9. Is appropriate action taken when the belongings of clients are lost or reported missing?

CLIENTS' MONEY

1. Do clients receive an adequate weekly income?
2. Are clients helped to appreciate the value of money and how to manage it?
3. Where appropriate, is a record kept of client finances?
4. Do clients receive their income or allowance in an individualised and dignified manner?
5. Where some discretion exists in client allowances, are clients involved in determining those amounts?
6. Do the more capable clients operate their own bank accounts?
7. Do clients have a safe and lockable place to keep their money?
8. Do clients have unrestricted access to their money?
9. Do clients have all the normal opportunities to spend their money?

10. Are clients free from having to purchase items which should be provided by the residence?
11. Is the residence free of punishment systems involving fines?
12. Is a client's permission obtained before his/her money is spent, used or saved?

SMOKING AND ALCOHOL

1. Are clients who are legally entitled to do so, free to smoke and drink if they wish to?
2. Is there a balance between the preferences of those who smoke and drink and those who do not?
3. Do helpers avoid using cigarettes as a form of manipulation?
4. Do helpers avoid imposing their personal standards on clients in relation to tobacco and alcohol use?
5. Does alcohol feature in a residence on social occasions?

RELATIONSHIPS

1. Are clients permitted to choose their own friends within and beyond the residence?
2. Are clients' friends taken into account when establishing living arrangements and routines?
3. Are clients supported in developing relationships?
4. Do helpers regard conversation between clients as private?
5. Do clients have plenty of opportunities to mix with people of both sexes?
6. Are clients able to entertain friends in private?
7. Do helpers accept that sexual interest and behaviour is as normal for disabled people as it is for others?
8. Is sex education available?
9. Do helpers encourage socially appropriate sexual behaviour in clients?
10. Do helpers behave in ways that make them appropriate models for clients?

11. Do helpers respect the privacy of clients in relation to the intimate aspects of their lives?
12. Is the residence sufficiently private and free from outside intrusion to enable normal relationships to develop?
13. Do helpers receive all necessary assistance to enable them to counsel, support and assist clients in developing and maintaining relationships?
14. Can clients discuss matters relating to sexuality and personal relationships in supportive contexts?
15. Is assistance available to clients who have very special problems in personal relationships?
16. Do helpers question their own moral values in terms of relevance for clients, and do they consciously avoid imposing them?

DAILY LIFE

1. Can the daily routine for clients be described as a normal one?
2. Are clients, within reason, free to get up and go to bed when they wish?
3. Are the basic aspects of the day, such as getting up in the morning, showering, using the toilet and going to bed, individualised?
4. Do clients receive the degree of help they need?
5. Are all efforts made to enable clients to determine and control their own daily routine?
6. Are the major events of the day consistent with client need?
7. Is there a different and more relaxed routine at weekends and on public holidays?
8. Are ritualistic aspects of the daily routine questioned and, where found to be inappropriate, modified?
9. Is the routine sufficiently flexible to accommodate unforseen events such as visitors?

10. Are helpers known by their names and not formal titles?
11. Do helpers wear everyday clothes?

MEALS

1. When menus are planned, are clients involved?
2. Do all clients eat in a dining room?
3. Do clients choose with whom they sit?
4. Are groups at tables less than eight?
5. Are mealtimes generally pleasant occasions?
6. Are clients able to eat their meals in an unhurried way?
7. Are clients encouraged to feed themselves?
8. Is the timing of the three main meals of the day appropriate?
9. Is there a mixture of formal, everyday and informal meals?
10. Are meals attractively presented, varied and well-balanced?
11. Are special diets provided for clients needing them?
12. Are individual food preferences recognised?
13. Can residents serve themselves at mealtimes?
14. Is food served at the correct temperature?
15. Is food available in sufficient quantities?
16. Is extra food available for second helpings?
17. Do staff sit at dining tables with clients and eat the same food?
18. Are clients encouraged to develop appropriate mealtime social graces?
19. Is appropriate cutlery and crockery used?
20. Are clients taught to use cutlery?
21. Are mealtimes flexible?
22. Can clients still have their meals if they are not on time?
23. Do helpers avoid imposing diets on clients?
24. Where possible, are clients involved in or do they actually prepare their own meals?
25. Are snacks available when clients need them?

26. Are clients able to prepare snacks for themselves between meals?

DOMESTIC WORK

1. Do clients have a choice as to whether they undertake chores beyond those which relate to their individual needs and immediate living situations?
2. Where clients spend the greater part of their day undertaking chores which relate to the maintenance of their residence, is this consistent with their individual plans?
3. Where clients work full-time on chores, do they receive appropriate payment?
4. Is the term therapy avoided in relation to domestic work?

SPECIAL OCCASIONS

1. Are the birthdays of clients remembered?
2. Are birthdays individually celebrated and in ways that are not institutional?
3. Do clients have a choice as to how their birthdays are celebrated?
4. Is Christmas celebrated in normal ways?
5. Are clients free from undue pressure to spend Christmas away from a residence?
6. Does the pattern and pace of life in the residence change in an appropriate way on public holidays?
7. Do clients have a holiday each year?

SMALL COMMUNITY RESIDENCES

1. Is there recognition of the need to develop small community residences?
2. Are helpers aware of what is involved in developing these residences?
3. Are small community residences appropriately sited?
4. Are suitable houses/flats selected as small community residences?
5. Are the close relatives of clients involved appropriately in the life of a residence?

6. Are residences flexibly staffed and according to client need?
7. Is an appropriate process used for the selection of clients for residences?
8. Are clients able to decide whether or not they wish to move to a residence and with whom?
9. Are attempts made to prepare clients for life in small community residences?
10. Do clients determine the basic pattern of their daily life in community residences?
11. Are clients given all necessary support when experiencing difficulties in adjusting to life in the residence?
12. Are helpers appropriately involved where difficulties occur with neighbours?
13. When vacancies occur, are clients and direct care workers involved in deciding on new members of the group?
14. Are direct care workers given all necessary support by senior workers?

FAMILY INVOLVEMENT

1. Do helpers recognise the reasons why family involvement is so important?
2. Do helpers display positive attitudes to the relatives of clients and seek to develop informal, supportive relationships with them?
3. Do helpers welcome the interest and encourage the involvement of relatives?
4. Do helpers receive guidance on working with families?
5. Do helpers attempt to gain an understanding of the life situations of relatives, the problems they encounter and the assistance they need?
6. Are all necessary steps taken to maintain appropriate contacts with close relatives?
7. Do helpers ensure that relatives receive appropriate information about clients?
8. Where appropriate, are relatives involved in decision-making processes concerning clients?
9. Are relatives welcomed and given pleasant hospitality when they visit a residence?

10. Are visiting arrangements informal, flexible and experienced as pleasurable by clients, relatives and helpers?
11. Do relatives have ready access to clients and helpers when they visit?
12. Are relatives able to:
    - meet clients in private if they so wish
    - move freely in the residence
    - talk to and spend time with other clients
    - take clients out
    - stay for meals or be accommodated overnight where they have travelled some distance to visit?
13. Are clients able to make regular visits home?
14. Is assistance with travel provided to enable clients to visit their homes?
15. Where necessary, are relatives taught how to maintain specific programs when clients are at home?
16. Do helpers contact relatives whose frequency of visiting has declined?
17. Are relatives informed when clients are sick or have been involved in an accident?

INTEGRATION INTO COMMUNITY LIFE

1. Are helpers aware of the necessity to take steps to integrate clients into community life?
2. Do helpers take all necessary action to achieve client integration?
3. Do helpers avoid taking clients out in large groups?
4. When clients are outside a residence, is everything done to ensure that they appear normal and are responded to appropriately?
5. Are clients taught behaviour appropriate to community life?
6. Are all vehicles used to transport clients free from signs by which they might be stigmatised?

OFFICIAL VISITORS

1. Are the needs of clients considered first whenever visitors to the residence are being considered?
2. Are direct care workers and clients involved in making decisions about visitors?
3. Are limits placed on groups of visitors?
4. Are visitors informed about what is expected of them?
5. Are visitors offered adequate hospitality?
6. Are attempts being made to phase out institutional practices such as open days and fetes?

VOLUNTEERS

1. Are helpers aware of the benefits that volunteers can bring to the residence?
2. Do helpers recognise that a volunteer program can be successful only where competent helpers give time to recruitment, selection, training, deployment and support of volunteers?
3. Are helpers realistic in their expectations of volunteers?
4. Are helpers aware of the many ways in which volunteers can assist a residence and clients?
5. Has one helper overall responsibility for volunteer programs?
6. Are a variety of approaches used when recruiting volunteers?
7. Do helpers use appropriate and effective processes when selecting volunteers?
8. Are volunteers given adequate training before becoming involved in the life of the residence?
9. Are volunteers provided with support once they have begun to be involved?
10. Are difficulties relating to volunteers dealt with on their merits and not from an assumption that volunteers are to blame?

THE NEEDS OF CHILDREN

1. Are residential facilities for children separate from those of adults?

2. Are children cared for in small family-type groups?
3. Is the pattern of life in a residence similar to that of children living in their own families?
4. Is there sufficient structure in the daily routine to give children a sense of security?
5. Do helpers meet the basic parenting needs of children, i.e.
   - physical care
   - emotional intimacy and affection
   - individual attention
   - security
   - socialisation
   - safety
   - play?
6. Are children taught, as a natural part of everyday life, basic self-help skills, for example:
   - dressing
   - toileting
   - eating
   - personal hygiene?
7. Are children encouraged to be involved in aspects of the daily routine, for example:
   - chores
   - shopping
   - meal preparation?
8. Do children have unrestricted access to age-appropriate toys and games that belong to them?
9. Do children have adequate outdoor playspace and equipment, for example, swings, bicycles, climbing frames?
10. Do children have unrestricted access to all parts of the residence?
11. Do helpers and children share special occasions, trips and outings?
12. Are children, wherever possible, integrated into normal schools?
13. Do staff assist children with their school work?
14. Are children provided with all the normal things associated with school, for example, uniforms, books and money for educational trips and activities?
15. Do staff establish helpful relationships with school personnel?
16. Do children have regular contact with their natural parents?
17. Do children receive special care when ill or distressed?
18. Do children receive pocket money or allowances to spend as they wish?
19. Do children visit local community resources, for example, cinemas, shops, libraries, social clubs, swimming and sports centres, banks, post offices, doctors and dentists?
20. Are children able to have and be responsible for pets?

THE NEEDS OF ADOLESCENTS

1. Are helpers working with adolescents aware of their needs?
2. Are adolescents given all opportunities to act in an increasingly independent way?
3. Do helpers refrain from being overly judgemental when adolescents display attitudes, tastes and fashion which to them seem outrageous or unacceptable?
4. Do helpers provide appropriate emotional support when adolescents are coming to terms with their disabilities?
5. Do helpers strive to ensure that disabled adolescents develop a self-concept that is not based on a sense of inferiority?
6. Do adolescents receive appropriate sex education?

THE NEEDS OF AGED PEOPLE

1. Do helpers avoid viewing aged people in terms of a stereotype?
2. Do helpers seek to provide a pattern of daily life for aged people that involves considerable activity, rather than subjecting them to a life of passivity?
3. Are the lives of aged people in the residence as normal as possible?
4. Are all necessary steps taken to eliminate inappropriate medical conceptions of aged people?

WORK

1. Do helpers recognise the importance of work for disabled people?
2. Where clients work full-time on maintenance tasks in a residence, do they do so out of choice, and are they paid an appropriate wage?
3. Do helpers actively seek to find appropriate jobs for disabled clients in normal work situations?
4. Are clients appropriately prepared when they are commencing their first jobs?
5. Is all necessary support given to clients once they are employed?
6. Do helpers assist those who are unemployed to find alternative activities which offer a sense of achievement and fulfilment?

LEISURE

1. Do helpers have full knowledge of the leisure resources in the local neighbourhood?
2. Do clients know what leisure activities are available?
3. Are clients free to decide their own leisure activities?
4. Are clients involved in decision-making about leisure activities, including trips, outings and holidays?
5. Are individual interests and hobbies catered for in the residence?
6. Are all leisure activities age appropriate?
7. Are helpers encouraged to extend their own leisure interests to clients?
8. Are clients involved in community-based leisure pursuits?
9. Do clients pursue leisure activities in the community only on an individual basis or in small groups of similarly disabled people?
10. Do helpers visit community resources to facilitate community integration by discussing the possibility of the involvement of disabled people?

11. Do staff members go with clients when necessary:
    - to provide transport
    - to demonstrate appropriate skills and behaviour
    - to give emotional support
    - for company and friendship?
12. Do clients have an annual holiday away from the residence?
13. Are holiday arrangements chosen by clients, varied and appropriate?

PROBLEM BEHAVIOUR

1. Do helpers have a clear understanding of what is and what is not age-appropriate behaviour?
2. Are clients taught age-appropriate behaviour?
3. Are helpers' expectations of client behaviour realistic?
4. Are helpers' expectations sufficiently flexible to suit individual clients?
5. Are helpers sufficiently patient and tolerant of clients?
6. Are clients socialised in a manner consistent with mainstream society?
7. Do helpers and clients work together to establish flexible and informal rules in the residence?

ROLE AND QUALITIES OF HELPERS

1. Are helpers familiar with contemporary approaches to disabled people and the philosophies on which they are based?
2. Do helpers strive for equality in their relationships with clients?
3. Do helpers acknowledge that they should be accountable to clients?
4. Do helpers involve clients in decision-making?
5. Do helpers, where necessary, act as advocates for clients?
6. Do helpers take on the role of key worker for individual clients?

7. Do helpers have a personal commitment to clients?
8. Do helpers individualise assistance to clients?
9. Do helpers monitor and evaluate their own feelings and professional behaviour?
10. Are helpers fully aware of the needs of clients?
11. Do helpers assist clients only in ways that are appropriate?
12. Do helpers have obvious worthwhile relationships with clients?

MANAGING RESIDENTIAL FACILITIES

1. Do senior workers understand the nature of the management task?
2. Are managers aware of factors within and beyond the organisation that affect what they do?
3. Are managers aware of management styles, and the strengths and weaknesses of different ways of dealing with workers and organisational issues?
4. Have managers considered what management style is appropriate for their organisation or work group?
5. Do managers work on developing an effective personal management style?
6. Have managers formulated a personal code of ethics to govern their dealings with workers?
7. Are there written conditions of service for the employment of helpers?
8. Are managers competent in staff recruitment and selection?
9. Is there an appropriate induction process for new helpers?
10. Do helpers say they receive all necessary support to work effectively?
11. Do managers and helpers recognise the need for teamwork?
12. Do managers assume the initiative in developing and maintaining teams?
13. Do managers continually evaluate the impact of their own performance on team members?

14. Do managers do all they can to develop the teamwork skills of team members?
15. Are managers effective in resolving difficulties and conflict within teams?
16. Are helpers involved in all decisions likely to affect them?
17. Do managers strive to communicate effectively with helpers and clients?
18. Are there effective communication networks?
19. Is there open communication between managers, helpers and clients?
20. Are there regular staff and team meetings?
21. Do all those attending staff meetings and client planning meetings consider them to be effective?
22. Are managers and helpers aware of the signs of stress?
23. Are managers and helpers aware of the factors that causes stress in residential situations?
24. Are managers and helpers aware that clients, as well as helpers, experience stress?
25. Are managers and helpers aware of the impact of stress on individuals, groups and organisations?
26. Do managers work imaginatively to reduce stress?
27. Are managers operating from realistic beliefs when they conclude a helper to be a problem?
28. When faced with a worker who is problematic, do managers explore all factors associated with his/her behaviour?
29. Do managers use professional approaches when taking action to deal with workers perceived as difficult?

CHANGE IN RESIDENTIAL SITUATIONS

1. Do managers understand why change is necessary in residential accommodation?
2. When managers attempt to bring about change, do they use appropriate and acceptable methods?
3. Do managers formulate rational proposals for change?

4. Are consultants used when necessary to assist groups of helpers to understand what is happening in the residence, and to bring about necessary change?
5. Are the reasons for staff resistance to change recognised and responded to appropriately?

STAFF TRAINING

1. Is there recognition of the need for all levels of worker to receive basic and ongoing training?
2. Does the organisation of which the residence is part, develop training programs for individual helpers?
3. Are helpers encouraged and supported to be involved in training programs, conferences, etc., beyond the residence?
4. Are helpers assisted financially to enable them to increase their knowledge and skills?

DUTY ROSTERS OF DIRECT CARE WORKERS

1. Are helpers in the residence, including senior workers, able to differentiate between staff-centred and client-centred rosters?
2. Do the hours of work of helpers reflect the needs of clients?
3. Are there sufficient numbers of staff to ensure that the residence is appropriately staffed at all times, particularly at busy periods?
4. Do helpers have adequate time off, and is it appropriately spaced?
5. Are helpers prevented from regularly changing their rosters where those changes are at the expense of clients?
6. Are helpers attached to particular residences or units on a permanent basis and not regularly moved around for organisational convenience or because of general staffing problems?

7. Is time set aside for meetings during the working hours of helpers?

BOARDS OF MANAGEMENT

1. Where appropriate, do residences have boards of management?
2. Do those boards have appropriate responsibilities?
3. Is membership of boards representative, in particular, are clients represented?
4. Is a time limit set on membership?
5. Is the board seen to be functioning effectively and in the interests of clients and helpers?
6. Are all members of boards in touch with clients and direct care workers?

ACCOUNTABILITY

1. Are helpers throughout the organisation or residence familiar with the reasons why they should be accountable for what they do?
2. Where appropriate, is contracting used to improve services?
3. Do helpers understand what is meant by advocacy?
4. Are citizen advocate programs available?
5. Does the role of helper involve an advocate dimension?
6. Do helpers recognise the need to respond objectively to complaints?
7. Does the organisation or residence have a documented complaints procedure?
8. Is a complaints procedure known to all involved in a residence?
9. When serious complaints are made, are they dealt with by helpers not involved in the residence in question?
10. Are clients satisfied with the quality of residential life?
11. Are direct care workers satisfied with the quality of client care?

Bibliography

Adams J D 1980 Understanding and managing stress: a workbook in changing lifestyles. University Associates, San Diego

Adams J D (ed) 1980 Understanding and managing stress: a book of readings. University Associates, San Diego

Albrecht G L (ed) 1976 The sociology of physical disability and rehabilitation. University of Pittsburg Press, Pittsburgh

American Association of Mental Deficiency 1975 Rights of mentally retarded persons: position papers of the American Association on Mental Deficiency. American Association of Mental Deficiency, Washington

Anderson D 1982 Social work and mental handicap. Macmillan, London

Anderson R, Greer J (eds) 1976 Educating the severely and profoundly retarded. University Park Press, Baltimore

Appolloni T, Cappuccilli J, Cooke T (eds) 1980 Achievements in residential services for persons with disabilities: towards excellence. University Park Press, Baltimore

Baker B L, Seltzer G B, Seltzer M M 1974 As close as possible: community residences for retarded adults. Little, Brown, Boston

Bamford T 1982 Managing social work. Tavistock, London

Barton R 1976 Institutional neurosis, 3rd edn. Wright, Bristol

Begab M, Richardson S (eds) 1975 The mentally retarded and society: a social science perspective. University Park Press, Baltimore

Bell L, Klemz A 1981 Physical handicap: a guide for the staff of social services departments and voluntary agencies. Woodhead-Faulkner, Cambridge, UK

Bernstein N R (ed) 1970 Diminished people: problems and care of the mentally retarded. Little, Brown, Boston

Blatt B, Kaplan F 1966 Christmas in purgatory. Allyn and Bacon, Boston

Blaxter M 1976 The meaning of disability: a sociological study of impairment. Heinemann, London

Bliss E 1976 Getting things done: the ABCs of time management. Macmillan, Melbourne

Blum J 1978 Pseudoscience and mental ability: the origins and fallacies of the IQ controversy. Monthly Review Press, New York

Boswell D, Wingrove J (eds) 1974 The handicapped person in the community. Tavistock, London

Boswell D M, Jaehig W B, Mittler P 1975 A handicapped identity. Open University Press, Milton Keynes, UK

Bradley V 1978 Deinstitutionalisation of developmentally disabled persons: a conceptual analysis and guide. University Park Press, Baltimore

Braginsky D, Braginsky B 1971 Hansels and Gretels: studies of children in institutions for the mentally retarded. Holt, Rinehart and Winston, New York

Brearley P, Hall F, Gutridge P, Jones G, Roberts G 1980 Admission to residential care. Tavistock, London

Brearley P, Black J, Gutridge P, Roberts G, Tarran E 1982 Leaving residential care. Tavistock, London

Brill N 1976 Teamwork: working together in the human services. Harper and Row, New York

Brown R I, Hughson E A 1980 Training of the developmentally handicapped adult. Charles C Thomas, Springfield, Illinois

Bruininks R, Meyers C, Sigford B, Lakin K (eds) 1981 Deinstitutionalization and community adjustment of mentally retarded people. American Association of Mental Deficiency, Washington DC

Burns T, Stalker G M 1961 The management of innovation. Tavistock, London

Buscaglia L 1975 The disabled and their parents: a counselling challenge. Charles B Slack, Thorofare, New Jersey

Carr J 1980 Helping your handicapped child: a step-by-step guide to everyday problems. Penguin, Harmondsworth, UK

Chartered Society of Physiotherapy 1980 Handling the handicapped: a guide to the lifting and movement of disabled people. Woodhead-Faulkner, Cambridge, UK

Cherington C, Dybwad G (eds) 1974 New neighbours: the retarded citizen in quest of home. President's Committee on Mental Retardation, Washington DC

Cherniss C 1980 Staff burnout: job stress in human services. Sage, Beverley Hills

Chinn P, Drew C, Logan D L 1979 Mental retardation: a lifecycle approach, 2nd edn. Mosby, St Louis

Cleland C 1978 Mental retardation: a developmental approach. Prentce-Hall, New Jersey

Cleland C, Swartz J 1982 Exceptionalities through the lifespan. Macmillan, New York

Clough R 1982 Residential work. Macmillan, London

Collins T, Bruce T 1984 Staff support and staff training. Tavistock, London

Combs A, Avila D, Purkey W 1971 Helping relationships: basic concepts for the helping professions. Allyn and Bacon, Boston

Connis R, Sowers J, Thompson L (eds) 1978) Training the mentally handicapped for employment. Human Sciences Press, New York

Conrad P, Schneider J 1980 Deviance and medicalization: from badness to sickness. Mosby, St Louis

Craft M, Craft A 1978 Sex and the mentally handicapped. Routledge and Kegan Paul, London

Crossley R, McDonald A 1980 Annie's coming out. Penguin, Melbourne

Cruzic K 1982 Disabled? Yes. Defeated? No: resources for the disabled and their families, friends and therapists. Prentice-Hall, New Jersey

Dartington T, Miller E, Gwynne G 1981 A life together: the distribution of attitudes around the disabled. Tavistock, London

Darvil C, Munday B (eds) 1984 Volunteers in the personal social services. Tavistock, London

Davis A 1981 The residential solution. Tavistock, London

Davis L 1982 Residential care: a community resource. Heinemann, London

De Graff A 1979 Attendees and attendants: a guidebook of helpful hints. College and University Personnel Associates, Washington DC

de la Cruz F, LaVeck G (eds) 1974 Human sexuality and the mentally retarded. Pergamon, Baltimore

Dunphy D 1981 Organisational change by choice. McGraw-Hill, Sydney

Dyer W 1977 Team building: issues and alternatives. Addison-Wesley, Reading, Mass

Edelwich J 1980 Burnout: stages in disillusionment in the helping professions. Human Sciences Press, New York

Edgerton R B 1967 The cloak of competence: stigma in the lives of the mentally retarded. University of California Press, Berkeley, California

Edgerton, R B 1979 Mental retardation. Fontana/Open Books, London

Etten G, Arkell C, Vanetten C 1980 The severely and profoundly handicapped: programs, methods and materials. Mosby, St Louis

Evans B, Waites B 1981 IQ and mental testing: an unnatural science and its social history. Macmillan, London

Fairweather G, Sanders D, Tornatzky L 1974 Creating change in mental health organizations. Pergamon, New York

Farber B 1968 Mental retardation: its social context and social consequences. Houghton-Miffin, Boston

Fischer J, Gochros H 1975 Planned behaviour change: behaviour modification in social work. Free Press, New York

Flynn J, Nitch K (eds) 1980 Normalisation, social integration, and community services. University Park Press, Baltimore

Francis D, Woodcock M 1975 People at work: a practical guide to organisational change. University Associates, La Jolla, California

Freidson E 1970 Professional dominance: the social structure of medicine. Aldine, Chicago

Freidson E 1970 Profession of medicine: a study of the sociology of applied knowledge. Dodd-Meade, New York

Gathercole C 1981 Group homes — staffed and unstaffed. British Institute of Mental Handicap, Kidderminster, UK

Gathercole C 1981 Leisure, social integration and volunteers. British Institute of Mental Handicap, Kidderminister, UK

Gathercole C 1981 The resettlement team. British Institute of Mental Handicap, Kidderminister, UK

Goffman E 1961 Asylums: essays on the social situations of mental patients and other inmates. Penguin, Harmondsworth, UK

Goffman E 1964 Stigma: notes on the management of spoiled identity. Penguin, Harmondsworth, UK

Gordon S 1974 Sexual rights for the people who happen to be handicapped. Syracruse University Press, Syracruse, New Jersey

Greengross W 1976 Entitled to love: the sexual and emotional needs of the handicapped. Malaby Press, London

Greer J, Anderson R, Odle S (eds) 1982 Strategies for helping severely and multiply handicapped citizens. University Park Press, Baltimore

Hale G (ed) 1979 The source book for the disabled. Paddington Press, London

Halpern J, Sackett K, Binner P, Mohr C 1980 The myths of deinstitutionalization: policies for the mentally retarded. Westview, Boulder, Colorado

Handy C 1976 Understanding organizations. Penguin, Harmondsworth, UK

Hannam C 1980 Parents and mentally handicapped children, 2nd edn. Penguin, Harmondsworth, UK

Hayes S, Hayes R 1982 Mental retardation: law, administration and policy. Law Book Co, sydney

Heddell F 1980 Accident of birth: aspects of mental handicap. BBC, London

Hirschberg G G, Lewis L, Vaughan P 1976 Rehabilitation: a manual for the care of the disabled elderly, 2nd end. L B Lippincott, Philadelphia

Hobbs H 1976 The futures of children. Jossey-Bass, San Francisco

Howard J, Strauss A 1975 Humanising health care. Wiley, New York

Hutchison P, Lord J 1979 Recreation integration: issues and alternatives in leisure services and community involvement. Leisurability Publications, Ottawa

Hutten J 1977 Short term contracts in social work. Routledge and Kegan Paul, London

Into the streets: a book by and for disabled people. 1981 Disability Resources Centre, Collingwood, Australia

Illich I et al 1977 Disabling professions. Boyans, London

Jaco E G (ed) 1972 Patients, physicians and illness. Free Press, New York

Jones H 1979 The residential community: a setting for social work. Routledge and Kegan Paul, London

Jones K 1975 Opening the door: a study of new policies for the mentally handicapped. Routledge and Kegan Paul, London

Jones L (ed) 1983 Reflections on growing up. The Council for Exceptional Children, Reston, Virginia

Katz A, Martin K 1982 A handbook of services for the handicapped. Greenwood Press, Westport, Connecticut

Katz E 1970 The retarded adult at home. Special Child Publications Inc, Seattle

Kenihan K 1981 How to be the parents of a handicapped child — and survive. Penguin, Ringwood, Australia

King R D, Raynes N V, Tizard J 1971 Patterns of residential care: sociological studies in institutions for handicapped children. Routledge and Kegan Paul, London

Kurtz R 1977 Social aspects of mental retardation. Lexington Books, Lexington, Mass.

Laura R S (ed) 1980 Problems of handicap. Macmillan, Melbourne

Levi L 1981 Preventing work stress. Addison-Wesley, Reading, Mass.

Lewis J, Lewis M 1977 Community counselling: a human services approach. Wiley, New York

Locker D 1983 Disability and disadvantage: the consequences of chronic illness. Tavistock, London

Loring J, Burn G (eds) 1975 Integration of handicapped children in society. Routledge and Kegan Paul, London

Mackenzie R 1972 The time trap. McGraw-Hill, New York

McCormack M 1979 Away from home: the mentally handicapped in residential care. Constable, London

McDaniel J W 1976 Physical disability and human behaviour. Pergamon, New York

McGregor D 1960 The human side of enterprise. McGraw-Hill, New York

McLaughlin P 1979 Guardianship of the person. National Institute of Mental Retardation, Downsview, Ontario

Marinelli R, Del Orto A (eds) 1977 The psychological and social impact of physical disability. Springer, New York

Marlett N J 1971 The adaptive functioning index. Vocational and Rehabilitation Research Institute, Calgary

Martin G, Pear J 1978 Behaviour modification: what it is and how to do it. Prentice-Hall, Englewoods Cliffs, New Jersey

Menolascino F J, Pearson P H (eds) 1974 Beyond the limits: innovations in services for the severely and profoundly retarded. Special Child Publications, Seattle

Mercer J R 1973 Labeling the retarded. University of California Press, Berkeley

Miller E J, Gwynne G V 1972 A life apart: a pilot study of residential institutions for the physically handicapped and the young chronic sick. Tavistock, London

Money T, Cole T, Chilopen R 1975 Sexual options for paraplegics and quadriplegics. Little, Brown, Boston

Morris P 1969 Put away: a sociological study of institutions for the mentally retarded. Routledge and Kegan Paul, London

Novak A, Heal L (eds) 1980 Integration of developmentally disabled individuals into the community. Paul Brooks, Baltimore

Oliver M 1983 Social work with disabled people. Macmillan, London

Ollerton Report 1982 Middle management in residential work. Residential Care Association, London

Oswin M 1971 the empty hours: a study of the weekend life of handicapped children in institutions. Allen Lane, London

Oswin M 1978 Children in long-stay hospitals. Spastics International Medical Publications,

Parsons T 1951 The social system. Free Press, Chicago

Paul J, Neufeld G, Pelosi J (eds) 1977 Child advocacy within the system. Saracuse University Press, Syracuse

Paul J (ed) 1981 Understanding and working with parents of children with special needs. Holt, Rinehart and Winston, New York

Paul J, Steadman D, Neufeld G 1977 Deinstitutionalization: program and policy development. Syracuse University Press, Syracuse

Payne M 1982 Working in teams. Macmillan, London

Pearson G 1975 The deviant imagination: psychiatry, social work and social change. Macmillan, London

Perske R 1980 New life in the neighbourhood: how persons with retardation or other disabilities can help make a good community better. Abington, Nashville

Pringle, M K 1974 The needs of children. Hutchinson, London

Resnick H, Patti R (eds) 1980 Change from within: humanising welfare organisations. Temple University Press, Philadelphia

Rettig E 1973 ABCs for parents. Associates for Behaviour Change, Van Nuys, California

Roarty J 1981 Captives of care. Hodder and Stoughton, Sydney

Roos, P, McCann B, Addison M (eds) 1980 Shaping the future: community-based residential services and facilities for mentally retarded people. University Park Press, Baltimore

Rosen M, Clark G, Kivitz M (eds) 1976 The history of mental retardation, University Park Press, Baltimore

Rosen M, Clark G, Kivitz M 1977 Habilitation of the handicapped: new dimensions in programs for the developmentally disabled. University Park Press, Baltimore

Roth W 1981 The handicapped speak. McFarland, Jefferson, North Carolina

Russo J 1980 Serving and surviving as a human service worker. Brooks/Cole, Monterey, California

Rothman D J 1971 The discovery of the asylum. Little, Brown, Boston

Ryan J, Thomas F 1980 The politics of mental handicap. Penguin, Harmondsworth, UK

Ryan W 1976 Blaming the victim. Vintage Books, New York

Safilios-Rothschild C 1970 The sociology and social psychology of disability and rehabilitation. Random House, New York

Scheerenberger R C 1976 Deinstitutionalization and institutional reform. Charles C Thomas, Springfield, Illinois

Schulman E 1980 Focus on the retarded adult: programs and services. Mosby, St Louis

Schur E M 1971 Labelling deviant behaviour. Harper and Row, New York

Schur E 1980 The politics of deviance. Prentice-Hall, New Jersey

Scott D 1981 'Don't mourn for me — organise . . .' The social and political uses of voluntary organisations. Allen and Unwin, Sydney

Scull A 1979 Museums of madness: the social

organisation of insanity in nineteenth century England. Penguin, Harmondsworth, UK

Scull A T 1984 Decarceration — community treatment and the deviant — a radical view, 2nd edn. Prentice-Hall, New Jersey

Seligman M 1975 Helplessness: on depression, development and death. Freeman, San Francisco

Shearer A 1981 Disability: whose handicap? Blackwell, Oxford

Silverman D 1970 The theory of organisations. Heinemann, London

Simon G (ed) 1980 Modern management of mental handicap: a manual of practice. MTP Press, Lancester

Simon G (ed) 1981 Local services for mentally handicapped people. British Institute of Mental Handicap, Kidderminster, UK

Stubbins J (ed) 1977 Social and psychological aspects of disability: a handbook for practitioners. University Park Press, Baltimore

Suelzle M, Keenan V 1980 Parents as advocates for handicapped children: untapped resources for social change in the 1980's. Illinois University, Chicago

Sunley R 1983 Advocacy today: a human service practitioner's handbook. Family Service, New York

Sussman M B (ed) 1965 Disability and social deviance. American Sociological Association, Washington

Tannenbaum R, Schmidt W 1958 How to chose a leadership pattern. Harvard Business Review, March–April

Telford C, Sawrey J 1977 The exceptional individual, 3rd edn. Prentice-Hall, New Jersey

Thomas D 1978 The social psychology of childhood disability. Methuen, London

Toplis E 1979 Provision for the disabled. Blackwell, Oxford

Toplis E 1982 Social response to handicap. Longman, London

Turnbull A P, Turnbull H R 1978 Parents speak out: views from the other side of the two way mirror. Merrill, Columbus, Ohio

Turnbull H (ed) 1981 The least restrictive alternative: principles and practice. American Association on Mental Deficiency, Washington DC

United Cerebral Palsy Association 1973 A bill of rights for the handicapped. Crusader 3: 1–6

United Nations 1975 General Assembly Resolution 3447 (xxx) Declaration on the rights of disabled persons. United Nations, New York 9:12

Walker A (ed) 1982 Community care: the family, the state and social policy. Blackwell and Robertson, Oxford

Walker J, Shea T 1980 Behaviour modification: a practical approach for educators. Mosby, St Louis

Walton R, Elliott D (eds) 1980 Residential care: a reader in current theory and practice. Pergamon, Oxford

Warham J 1977 An open case: the organizational context of social work. Routledge and Kegan Paul, London

Warshaw L 1979 Managing stress. Addison-Wesley, Reading, Mass.

Wehman P 1981 Competitive employment: new horizons for severely disabled individuals. Paul Brooks, Baltimore

Whelan E, Speake B 1979 Learning to cope. Souvenir Press, London

Whittaker J 1979 Caring for troubled children. Jossey-Bass, San Francisco

Wilding P 1982 Professional power and social welfare. Routledge and Kegan Paul, London

Wilkin D 1979 Caring for the mentally handicapped child. Croom Helm, London

Wilson M 1979 Effective management of volunteer programs. Johnson, Colorado

Wing J, Olsen R (eds) 1979 Community care for the mentally disabled. Oxford University Press, Oxford

Wolfensberger W 1972 The principle of normalization in human services. National Institute of Mental Retardation, Toronto

Woodcock, M 1979 Team development manual. Gower Press, Aldershot, UK

Wright G 1980 Total rehabilitation. Little, Brown, Boston

Yule W, Carr J (eds) 1980 Behaviour modification for the mentally handicapped. Croom Helm, London

Index